The
LDN
Book 4

Chronic Pain
Case Studies

Low Dose Naltrexone-

EDITED BY LINDA ELSEGOOD

Printed in the United Kingdom

First printed April 2025

ISBN: 978-1-7391070-6-2

Published by LDN Research Trust

PO Box 1083

Buxton

Norwich

NR10 5WY

UK

www.ldnresearchtrust.org

PRAISE FOR THE LDN BOOK 4

A Game-Changer for Chronic Conditions. If you or a loved one has struggled with autoimmune diseases or chronic pain that hasn't responded to conventional treatments, this book is essential reading. It is well-researched. It explores the transformative potential of LDN, a safe and affordable therapy that has helped many regain their quality of life. With clear explanations, real-life case studies, and a strong scientific foundation, it makes a compelling case for LDN in managing conditions like multiple sclerosis, fibromyalgia, lupus, and more. Highly recommended for patients and healthcare providers.

Jay Watts RPh, FACA

This book deepens my appreciation for LDN and boosts my confidence as a practitioner. It highlights positive outcomes in treating conditions such as pain, autoimmune disorders like rheumatoid arthritis and multiple sclerosis, and paediatric issues such as juvenile idiopathic arthritis.

I have prescribed LDN for nearly a decade to patients of all ages—starting from as young as 8 months—including those suffering from PANS/PANDAS, Lyme disease, mold exposure, and chronic pain. Given its capacity to restore health, I believe LDN should be considered a first-line therapy for all healthcare practitioners.

Taylor Bean, ND, FMAPS

This book offers a compelling overview of the therapeutic potential of low-dose naltrexone (LDN) for various conditions that I encounter in my practice, including autoimmune diseases and chronic pain. It is a valuable resource for healthcare professionals and researchers, presenting scientific insights and clinical case studies.

Jonathan Kalman, NMD

The 4th book in this series presents cases of complex multisystem disorders that commonly confound and frustrate doctors and how the inclusion of LDN transformed their health even when things appeared hopeless.

In my practice, I saw many patients with such conditions. LDN rapidly became such an essential tool in my practice that I wish I'd discovered it at the start of my career.

All GPs should read these books. They prompt careful assessments of complex conditions and their aetiologies. With LDN's safety and flexible dosing, practitioners should consider integrating LDN into treatment plans, supported by the LDN Research Trust.

Philip Bradfield Stowell, MB BS (London)
FACNEM, GP Retired

This is another incredible book highlighting the many benefits of LDN, particularly in pain management. LDN has been a game changer for many patients who come to our pharmacy after being told their blood work is normal, yet they still don't feel well. We have always dispensed medication, but with LDN in our toolkit, we are offering hope. Thank you, Linda, for yet another fantastic book.

Steve Irsfeld, RPh

The results of LDN have been impressive, as illustrated in this book. It's disappointing that Big Pharma tends to overlook it due to a lack of financial incentive. Yet, many individuals facing health challenges have improved their lives with LDN, finding renewed hope for well-being. When I faced fibromyalgia and chronic pain in 1996, I would have embraced the chance to regain my health through monitored LDN titration with a qualified practitioner. This approach might have spared me the long journey to recovery that I ultimately had to undertake.

Marlene Kennedy, GCFP

Dedication

To those who bravely navigate the stuggles of chronic pain, may you find the answers and strength you seek.

Contents

Foreword

History of Naltrexone and the Emergence of Low-Dose Use

Pradeep Chopra, MD

Naltrexone was first synthesized in the 1960s and approved by the U.S. Food and Drug Administration (FDA) in 1984 as a treatment for opioid addiction. Initially used at doses of 50 mg to 100 mg per day, naltrexone functions as an opioid antagonist, blocking the effects of opioids like heroin or morphine and helping individuals overcome addiction. It later gained FDA approval for the management of alcohol dependence, where it reduces cravings and consumption.

The concept of low-dose naltrexone (LDN) emerged in the 1980s, pioneered by Dr Bernard Bihari, a New York-based physician. Dr Bihari hypothesized that administering naltrexone in doses much lower than those used for addiction—typically 1.5 mg to 4.5 mg—could modulate the immune system. This led to a surge in interest in its off-label use in various chronic and autoimmune conditions, sparking research and anecdotal reports of success.

Low-dose naltrexone (LDN) is a modified version of Naltrexone, a medication traditionally used in higher doses to manage opioid and alcohol dependence. However, in significantly lower doses, LDN has shown promise in managing a range of chronic conditions, including autoimmune diseases, inflammatory disorders, and even certain cancers. This article will delve into the mechanism, potential benefits, side effects, and practical considerations of LDN to provide a thorough understanding of its therapeutic potential.

Understanding Naltrexone and Low Dose Naltrexone (LDN)
Naltrexone is an opioid receptor antagonist, meaning it blocks opioid receptors in the brain, which helps to reduce cravings and dependency on opioids or alcohol. In traditional doses (usually 50 mg or more), it is primarily used to treat addiction. However, in much smaller doses, typically between 0.5 and 4.5 mg daily, it works differently in the body, showing immune-modulating effects that can benefit a broader range of conditions.

Mechanism of Action
Naltrexone, even at low doses, works primarily as an antagonist to opioid receptors, including the mu-opioid receptor (MOR), kappa-opioid receptor (KOR), and delta-opioid receptor (DOR). Its mechanism in low doses differs substantially from its use in addiction treatment. The key actions include:

- Transient Opioid Receptor Blockade: When LDN is taken, it temporarily blocks opioid receptors for a few hours. This short-term blockade leads to a positive biofeedback effect that increases the production of endogenous opioids, such as beta-endorphins and enkephalins. These molecules play a crucial role in reducing pain and inflammation and promoting a sense of well-being.

- Immune Modulation: LDN influences the immune system by reducing the activity of microglia, the resident immune cells of the central nervous system. Overactive microglia can release inflammatory cytokines, contributing to chronic pain and neuroinflammation. By modulating this activity, LDN may help reduce inflammation.

- Toll-Like Receptor (TLR) Antagonism: Naltrexone inhibits Toll-like receptor 4 (TLR4), a key immune system component in producing inflammatory cytokines. This action contributes to its potential role in autoimmune and inflammatory diseases.

Toll-like receptors (TLRs) are a family of pattern recognition receptors (PRRs) that play a fundamental role in the innate immune system. They recognize molecular patterns associated with pathogens (pathogen-associated molecular patterns, PAMPs) and endogenous signals released during tissue damage (damage-associated molecular patterns, DAMPs). TLRs activate signaling cascades that orchestrate inflammatory responses, bridging innate and adaptive immunity. While TLRs are crucial for defense against infections, their dysregulation is implicated in various pathological conditions, including chronic pain. Emerging evidence suggests that TLR-mediated inflammation contributes to central and peripheral sensitization, key mechanisms underlying chronic pain syndromes.

- Enhancing Cellular Repair: Opioid growth factors (OGFs), primarily met-enkephalin, are endogenous peptides that regulate cell growth and immune modulation. Unlike classical opioid peptides that mainly mediate pain relief by acting on opioid receptors in the nervous system, OGFs exert their effects by binding to the opioid growth factor receptor (OGFr). This interaction is crucial in regulating cell proliferation, immune function, and inflammation.

OGFs maintain homeostasis in various tissues, influencing wound healing, immune responses, and neuroprotection processes. By modulating these pathways, OGFs have been implicated in managing chronic pain, autoimmune conditions, and certain cancers.

Low-dose naltrexone (LDN) has been studied for its unique mechanism in modulating the opioid growth factor (OGF)–opioid growth factor receptor (OGFr) axis, which plays a critical role in cell growth regulation and immune modulation. Unlike its conventional use as an opioid antagonist, LDN at low doses (typically 1.5–4.5

mg) works by transiently blocking opioid receptors, leading to a compensatory upregulation of endogenous opioids, including OGF (also known as met-enkephalin) and an increase in OGFr expression.

This enhanced OGF–OGFr interaction has been shown to regulate inflammation, promote tissue repair, and modulate immune function, key factors in chronic pain conditions such as fibromyalgia, complex regional pain syndrome, and neuropathic pain. Additionally, LDN's effects on microglial activation in the central nervous system contribute to its ability to reduce neuroinflammation, further supporting its role as a novel therapy for chronic pain management.

Overall, LDN's modulation of the OGF–OGFr pathway represents a promising non-opioid approach to chronic pain, offering potential benefits with a low side-effect profile and minimal risk of dependency compared to traditional opioid treatments.

Conditions that May Benefit from LDN
Autoimmune Diseases:
LDN has been explored as a treatment for several autoimmune conditions, including:

- Multiple Sclerosis (MS): Many patients with MS report symptom improvement with LDN. It is thought to reduce inflammation and neurodegeneration associated with the disease.
- Rheumatoid Arthritis: Patients with rheumatoid arthritis may find relief as LDN can decrease joint inflammation.
- Lupus, Crohn's disease, and Ulcerative Colitis: LDN has shown promise in gastrointestinal and connective tissue autoimmune diseases by modulating the immune response.

Chronic Pain Disorders:
- Patients with fibromyalgia, chronic fatigue syndrome, and complex regional pain syndrome have reported reduced pain

and better sleep quality with LDN. The medication may decrease neuroinflammation and help regulate the central nervous system's pain processing.

Cancer:
- Preliminary studies suggest that LDN may inhibit tumor growth by modulating the immune system, enhancing the body's ability to target cancer cells. LDN is not a cure for cancer, but some oncologists use it as a supportive therapy.

Mental Health and Neurodegenerative Disorders:
- Because of its potential effects on the central nervous system, LDN is being studied in Alzheimer's disease, Parkinson's disease, and depression.

Skin Conditions:
- Reports show improvement in patients with psoriasis and eczema. LDN's anti-inflammatory properties help alleviate symptoms associated with these skin disorders.

Benefits of Low-Dose Naltrexone
- Reduced Inflammation: By modulating immune response, LDN can help reduce systemic inflammation, benefiting conditions like arthritis and inflammatory bowel disease.
- Minimal Side Effects: Compared to traditional treatments, LDN is generally well-tolerated and has fewer side effects.
- Non-Addictive: As an opioid antagonist, LDN does not create dependence, making it a safer long-term option.
- Affordable: LDN is relatively inexpensive, often making it an accessible treatment option.

Possible Side Effects and Risks

While LDN is generally well-tolerated, some patients may experience mild side effects, especially during the initial stages of treatment. Common side effects include:

- Sleep Disturbance: Insomnia or vivid dreams can occur initially.
- Gastrointestinal Issues: Some patients report mild nausea or stomach discomfort.
- Headaches may occur in a small percentage of users, often dissipating after a few weeks.

These side effects are usually mild and transient; adjusting the dosage can often mitigate them.

Dosage and Administration

The recommended dosage of low-dose naltrexone (LDN) varies based on the treated condition and the individual patient's response. Typically, the dosing ranges between 0.5 to 4.5 mg daily, although some patients may start at lower doses to assess their tolerance. There have been anecdotal reports of patients responding to doses of up to 10 mg of LDN daily.

Practical Considerations:

- Monitoring and Adjustments: Monitoring symptoms and adjusting the dose based on tolerance and effectiveness is essential. Patients should work closely with their healthcare provider. One such example would be in the management of Hashimoto's thyroiditis. Patients treated with LDN for Hashimoto's thyroiditis should monitor their thyroid function.
- Possible Drug Interactions: While rare, LDN can interact with opioid-based medications.

Conclusion

Low-dose naltrexone offers a potential therapeutic option for those struggling with autoimmune diseases, chronic pain, and certain mental health conditions. Its role as a disease modifying agent in most conditions, its low cost, low side effect profile, and potential benefits make it a valuable treatment.

Autoimmune and Inflammatory Diseases

Holistic Approaches to Severe Arthritis and Epilepsy

Rehana Sajjad, MD, FACOG, ABAARM

Abstract

This case study examines the management of severe arthritis pain and epilepsy in a 68-year-old female patient. Alongside her increasing and immobilizing pain, her epileptic seizures were becoming more frequent. SM came to see me searching for help as her life was becoming unbearable. A comprehensive treatment plan, including low-dose naltrexone (LDN), peptides, and lifestyle changes, helped to reduce inflammation, thereby improving her mobility, reducing her pain, and reducing the frequency of her epileptic seizures.

Introduction

Inflammation and pain lead to stress, prompting the body to release chemicals that increase inflammation. This heightened inflammation can cause more pain, stiffness, and possible joint damage in inflammatory arthritis conditions like rheumatoid arthritis (RA), psoriatic arthritis (PsA), and ankylosing spondylitis (AS). Additionally, the psychological effects of managing arthritis, which can be both painful and persistent, often raise stress levels. This, in turn, can further aggravate the condition, creating a cycle of worsening symptoms.

Inflammation has a complex and significant role in epilepsy, possibly aiding in the initiation and recurrence of seizures, as well as the development of the condition itself (epileptogenesis). It affects neuronal excitability, compromises brain tissue integrity, and alters synaptic functioning. Stress is often recognized as a seizure trigger for individuals with epilepsy. It can exacerbate anxiety and trigger hormone release that affects brain function, which may lead to seizures.

Patient Description

SM is a 68-year-old female patient from Pakistan. She is struggling with her mobility due to pain and inflammation negatively impacting her life, and her epileptic seizures are becoming more frequent as the stress of her situation intensifies. Furthermore, she faces financial difficulties that have restricted her access to essential lab work and conventional medical treatments.

History

Patient SM presented with severe bilateral knee joint pain, which she described as "extremely intense." Additionally, she reported an increase in both the frequency and severity of her epileptic seizures. The pain significantly impacted her mobility, making it difficult for her to walk and affecting her overall sleep quality. Her quality of life was poor.

Treatment Plan

As a holistic physician, a comprehensive treatment plan was developed, incorporating dietary modifications, nutritional supplementation, and alternative therapies aimed at alleviating inflammation and pain and managing her epilepsy.

- Dietary Adjustments: The elimination of gluten, sugar, and dairy products was recommended to reduce inflammation and enhance overall health.
- Alternative Therapies - low-dose naltrexone (LDN): Administered at a dose of 1.5 mg daily to help manage pain and inflammation.
- Nutritional Supplements: Peptides: Including TB4 Active Fragment and KPV to support healing and recovery, Curcumin:

Incorporated for its well-known anti-inflammatory properties, Vitamins: Vitamin D, K2, multivitamins, Vitamin C, and magnesium to address potential deficiencies and support general health.

- Therapeutic Measures: Epsom salt baths were advised to promote relaxation and alleviate muscular pain. Red light and near-infrared therapy were administered using a cap designed for the head and knees, aimed at reducing inflammation and enhancing tissue repair.

Expected Outcome

We aimed to lower inflammation, which could alleviate pain and, in the process, decrease stress, ultimately reducing the frequency of her epilepsy.

Actual Outcome

Regular follow-up communications were maintained with the patient following the implementation of the treatment plan. Over time, patient SM reported significant improvements:

- She became pain-free and expressed satisfaction regarding her recovery.
- Her mobility improved, allowing her to resume daily activities independently.
- The frequency of her epileptic seizures decreased, indicating better control over her condition.

The patient is considering knee joint replacement surgery to improve her mobility and quality of life further.

Conclusion

This case illustrates the efficacy of a holistic approach to managing complex health issues such as severe arthritis and epilepsy. Through dietary changes, nutritional supplements, and alternative therapies, significant advancements in pain management and seizure control were achieved, enabling the patient to contemplate further medical interventions for her joint health. Ongoing monitoring and support remain essential for sustaining her well-being and addressing her continuous health concerns.

Juvenile Idiopathic Arthritis

Edyta Biernat-Kaluza MD, PhD

Abstract
A 10-year-old boy with congenital toxoplasmosis presented with pain in both hands and wrists, accompanied by morning stiffness, at an orthopedic office. The physical examination revealed a diminished range of motion (ROM) in the right wrist. After one month, the symptoms worsened, and he was diagnosed with juvenile idiopathic arthritis (JIA). Methotrexate combined with steroid therapy was recommended, but the parents only consented to the steroids. They began exploring alternative/complementary management options, including CBD, a nonpharmacological approach, and low-dose naltrexone (LDN).

LDN was administered orally (starting with a daily dose of 0.2 mg) and topically. Simultaneously, systemic deflazacort (instead of prednisone) was gradually reduced. His clinical condition improved significantly: the range of motion in his wrists and hands normalized, and laboratory abnormalities were also corrected. Currently, he is taking 3 mg of LDN both orally and topically. The holistic approach, including LDN treatment with vitamin D3, probiotics, mitoceuticals, and an anti-inflammatory diet, has successfully achieved remission of JIA alongside a history of lambliasis and resolved Chlamydia/ Mycoplasma pneumonia infections.

Introduction
Juvenile idiopathic arthritis (JIA) is a serious chronic condition and one of the most common disabling disorders in children under 16 years, with seven distinct subtypes. The persistence of symptoms— swelling and/or pain along with restricted movement—lasting beyond six weeks confirms the objective presence of arthritis.

A delay in diagnosis may lead to irreversible changes, not only in the musculoskeletal system but also beyond. Furthermore, interdisciplinary healthcare professionals, including rheumatologists, ophthalmologists, endocrinologists, physiotherapists, and others, should be involved in the treatment of JIA. Treatment typically begins with NSAIDs, followed by glucocorticoids, and the best options include ultrasound-guided intraarticular injections. Systemic steroids should be avoided due to their widely recognized adverse effects, which, in children, may additionally cause growth suppression.

A serious complication of disease activity may involve facial deformities resulting from severe retrognathism, often referred to as a "bird-like" face. The next step in treatment includes slow-acting anti-rheumatic drugs such as methotrexate, sulfasalazine, hydroxychloroquine, and various biological agents (for example, anti-TNF) or newer JAK inhibitors. However, the most significant concern is pain. Given the anti-inflammatory and analgesic properties of low-dose naltrexone (LDN), which has minimal side effects, it should be considered for patients with JIA. (EULAR Textbook on the Rheumatic Diseases; Editor Johannes WJ Bijlsma; 2012; BMJ Group)

Patient Description
A 10-year-old boy was born in the first critical care unit with congenital toxoplasmosis. His mother received Rovamycin during the third trimester, and Sulfadiazine was administered to the boy for his first year of life.

Case History
At the beginning of January 2022, the boy woke up with pain and contractures in both hands and wrists, especially the right one, accompanied by morning stiffness. His mother suspected that the symptoms resulted from playing a video game console for about

1.5 hours per day over the previous six weeks. During the physical exam, the orthopedic surgeon who examined the boy found a reduced range of motion (ROM) in the right wrist. Additionally, he noted a slouching tendency and head anteversion. An ultrasound examination revealed a small effusion and bilateral tendonitis of the second extensor thumb (similar to psoriatic arthritis). The only abnormality in the laboratory tests was elevated transaminases. The orthopedic recommendations included a hepatological consultation and locally administered NSAIDs, topical ice treatment, and exercises to improve the ROM of the right wrist. If there was no improvement, physiotherapist-conducted rehabilitation was advised.

After one month and a deterioration of symptoms, the boy was consulted by a pediatric rheumatologist who diagnosed him with JIA and recommended methotrexate with steroid therapy. However, the parents did not want to start this type of immunotherapy and only accepted steroid treatment. They began to look for alternative/complementary management options. The boy was then seen by an ophthalmologist, who found no abnormalities. Next, he met with a pediatric specialist, and intermittent CBD (without THC) therapy was initiated. Thanks to this, the boy's energy and sleep quality improved significantly. One month before his visit to my office, he reported stomach pain. I first saw the patient at the end of February 2022.

Physical Examination
During physical examination, bilaterally, pain, edema, and limited range of movement of both wrists/hands, especially right, were stated. Although he has taken prednisone 5 mg orally for one month, he was practically unable to move his wrists due to edema; this time, ultrasound confirmed tendonitis in both, particularly in the right wrist and metacarpals. Other signs and symptoms included a small right knee effusion, which was confirmed by ultrasound examination.

Test Results
Abnormalities February 2022:
- Thrombocytes: 431 n <400
- Eosinophilia: 9% n <5%
- AspAt: 55 n <40
- ALAT: 62 n <40
- Vitamin D3 25(OH): 23 ng/ml
- D-dimer: 2.27 n <0.5
- ANA positive: 1:160
- Anti-Giardia lamblia IgM: 1:32 elevated
- Anti-chlamydia pneumoniae IgM and IgA: elevated
- Anti-Mycoplasma pneumoniae IgM and IgA: elevated

Moreover:
- RF: negative
- Anti-CCP: negative
- HLA B27 and Cw6 genes: not present

During the Last Consultation:
- Thrombocytes: 361
- Eosinophilia: 11.3% n <5%
- Vitamin D3 25(OH): 66.4 ng/ml
- D-dimer: 0.36 n <0.5
- AspAt: 33 n <40
- ALAT: 22 n <40

Diagnosis:
- Juvenile idiopathic arthritis - JIA subtype - oligoarthritis
- Vitamin D3 deficiency
- Lambliosis
- Congenital Toxoplasmosis

- Reactive arthritis due to Chlamydia and Mycoplasma pneumoniae infections

Treatment Plan

Initially, I switched from prednisone 5 mg to deflazacort 6 mg (which leads to fewer adverse events), recommended US-guided steroid intra-articular injections (commonly referred to as blockades), and suggested LDN treatment. A non-pharmacological approach was taken, which involved a nutritional anti-inflammatory elimination diet based on IgG food intolerances, along with physiotherapy for range of motion (ROM). At first, topical LDN ointment was prescribed. An initial oral dose of LDN 0.2 mg was recommended during the next visit. Later, the oral dose of LDN was increased to 0.5 mg, with a suggestion to raise the dosage by 0.2 mg every 10 days until reaching 10% of his body weight, which was 2.2 mg at that point.

After six months of LDN treatment, the boy gained weight and reached an oral dose of 2.5 mg. He continued using LDN topically as well. Gradually, we observed improvements in clinical, laboratory, and ultrasound findings. Concurrently, he has been prescribed antibiotics (initially clarithromycin, later azithromycin) due to reactive arthritis following a past Chlamydia pneumonia infection. Later, he was unable to continue Salazopyrin EN due to an allergy to salicylates. The patient also continued with CBD + CBG 10% therapy. Thanks to the holistic approach involving LDN treatment, he was able to stop taking steroids in the summer of 2024.

Currently, the oral dose of LDN is 3 mg. Due to rising eosinophilia, he was referred for parasitic diagnostics.

Expected Outcome

The expectation was reduced inflammation and pain, improving the patient's condition overall. This would result in less joint stiffness and greater mobility.

Actual Outcome

During the last phone consultation in November 2024, his mother reported that the patient was in excellent condition, pain-free, and weighing 30 kg. The boy plays the drums without any deterioration in his wrists. Additionally, the parents were pleased that he no longer had to take steroids.

Conclusion

LDN therapy should be regarded as a highly effective option for children with JIA, particularly in instances involving accompanying pain. (Theriault, Omonike Oyelola, and Zempsky 2023; Karlo Toljan and Bruce Vrooman 2018; Jarred Younger, Luke Parkitny, and David McLain 2014; Norman Brown, Jaak Panksepp 2009; Jarred Younger et al., 2013; Phillip S. Kim and Michael A. Fishman 2020).

Transformative Management of Psoriatic Arthritis

Edyta Biernat-Kaluza MD, PhD

Abstract

A 65-year-old woman, after undergoing two neurosurgical operations for lumbar and cervical spine stabilization, was referred to a rheumatological outpatient clinic by her neurosurgeon for diagnosis and treatment. She reported experiencing intense calf pain since childhood. While the sciatica pain resolved following the surgery, she continued to suffer from severe pain in the coccyx and ischial tuberosities. Rheumatological diagnostics revealed psoriatic arthritis and a comprehensive treatment plan was initiated, which included dietary changes, vitamin D3, probiotics, and other supplements.

The primary therapy involved low-dose naltrexone (LDN), beginning with a dose of 0.5 mg and increasing by 0.5 mg every 10 days. After 16 months, she reached her "happy dose" of 1 mg in the morning and 4.5 mg in the evening. As a result, she can now walk 7 kilometers without any decline in her condition. No immunosuppressive therapy is necessary. For her, LDN therapy has been a "game changer" in managing her illness and enhancing her quality of life. Thanks to the LDN therapy, she feels very well and reports no pain. Her quality of life has improved significantly.

Introduction

Psoriatic arthritis (PsA) is a chronic, seronegative arthritis characterized by the absence of rheumatoid factor (RF-). It is classified within a group known as spondyloarthropathies (SpA). SpA typically occurs in genetically predisposed individuals, particularly those with the genes HLAB27 and/or HLA Cw6.

Key features of PsA include involvement of the synovium, entheses, and extra-articular sites. Enthesitis refers to inflammation at the entheses, where tendons, ligaments, fascia, or joint capsules attach to bone. The most common extra-articular manifestation is psoriasis, which can affect the skin and nails. A family history of psoriasis in first or second-degree relatives can also be significant for diagnosis.

Diagnosing PsA can be challenging because there are no definitive laboratory tests. Therefore, detecting the presence of the gene HLA-Cw6 is crucial, as it can help identify both psoriasis and psoriatic arthritis. The CASPAR (Classification Criteria for Psoriatic Arthritis) criteria facilitate the diagnosis; a patient is considered to have psoriatic arthritis if they score at least 3 points.

Early diagnosis of PsA and the initiation of effective treatment are essential, as the disease's natural progression can lead to disability, reduced quality of life, and various complications, including cardiovascular issues, eye inflammation, and fractures due to osteoporosis.

First-line treatment for PsA typically involves nonsteroidal anti-inflammatory drugs (NSAIDs), followed by disease-modifying anti-rheumatic drugs (DMARDs) such as methotrexate, sulfasalazine, or leflunomide. Biologics, including anti-TNF-alpha blockers, anti-IL-23 blockers, anti-IL-17A inhibitors, and a newer class known as JAK inhibitors, are the most effective options in classical rheumatology.

Rehabilitation is also a crucial component of managing PsA. (EULAR Textbook on Rheumatic Diseases, 2015).

Patient Description
A 65-year-old woman was referred to my rheumatology office in July 2022 by a neurosurgeon for diagnosis and treatment. She reported experiencing intense calf pain since childhood. Later, during her two pregnancies, she suffered severe pain similar to sciatica. Five years ago, her lower back pain became more pronounced.

She is very sensitive to cold and has required treatment at a pain clinic, where she was prescribed baclofen, gabapentin, and even buprenorphine patches.

Due to severe spinal pain, the patient underwent two neurosurgical operations: stabilization of the lumbar vertebrae (L4/L5) and a similar procedure on her cervical spine. While her sciatica initially improved after the surgeries, she continued to experience intense pain, particularly in the coccyx and ischial tuberosity regions. Six months before her referral to the rheumatologist, she received ultrasound-guided steroid injections in these areas and again five months before the referral. These procedures were complicated by trembling and an increase in calf contracture.

Despite the neurosurgical operations, she is unable to walk long distances due to severe pain in both thighs, the sacral area, and the ischial tuberosities. She has been using NSAIDs, specifically coxibs, such as etoricoxib 90 mg, on a chronic basis. Additionally, she has a history of transient skin psoriasis and has experienced kidney stones on two occasions.

History
Her pain is primarily in the tendons, especially at the entheses around the knee joints (right side more than left). She reported experiencing intense pain in her buttocks every early morning around 4 AM, which is characteristic of inflammatory back pain (IBP) and typical of spondyloarthropathies. During the first consultation, I decided to conduct a differential diagnosis to specifically rule out a purely spondyloarthropathic background. Tests were ordered for HLA genes, specifically loci B and Cw6.

She was quite surprised to learn that the cause of her condition and pain could be psoriatic arthritis (PsA), as indicated by the presence of the HLA-Cw6 gene. This revelation jogged her memory of experiencing transient skin psoriasis in the past. Additionally, there is a positive family history, as her uncle (her father's brother) suffers from skin psoriasis.

Physical Examination

Her body weight was 70 kg, and her height was 164 cm. She experienced some difficulty walking. During the physical examination, the following findings were noted:
- Contractures in both knee joints, particularly in the right knee
- Painful entheses around both knees
- Pain localized at both ischial tuberosities
- Discomfort in the coccyx area
- Sensitivity of the pubic symphysis upon palpation
- Painful muscles in both calves

Additionally, cold feet were observed, but there were no signs of Raynaud's phenomenon or livedo reticularis. No skin or nail psoriasis was present.

Test Results
- Fibrynogen 394 mg/dl n< 350 mg/dl
- Vitamin B12 166 pg/ml n: 187-883 pg/ml
- Homocysteine 13,4 umol/ml preferable <10 umol/ml
- DHEA-S 12,6 ug/dl (29,7-260) ug/dl
- HLA-B27 negative
- HLA-Cw6 positive
- MRI of the pelvis in September 2022 revealed enthesopathy without active features and pubic symphysis narrowing.

She had 3 points of CASPAR criteria:
- History of psoriasis (in the absence of current psoriasis) 1 point
- A family history of psoriasis in the second degree relative to 1 point

- Rheumatoid factor negativity 1 point

Diagnosis
- Psoriatic arthritis in a person with the presence of Cw6 gene
- Vitamin D3 deficiency in the past
- Vitamin B12 deficiency
- Kidney stones
- Stabilization of lumbar and cervical spine
- Advanced osteopenia

Treatment Plan and Progression

In the beginning, magnesium was administered orally and transdermally (in oil and Epsom salt baths). After obtaining laboratory tests and genetic testing results, I recommended a dietary change to eliminate "inflammatory" foods and those based on IgG food intolerance due to autoimmune reasons. Simultaneously, she received calcifediol, catalpa, a homocysteine-reducing supplement, butyric acid, probiotics, and mitoceutics such as CoQ10 and glutathione. She was also offered low-dose naltrexone (LDN) treatment and received informational leaflets about it. In August 2022, she began using LDN, starting at a dose of 0.5 mg, which was increased by 0.5 mg every 10 days. By March 2023, she could walk 7 km without any pain. In May 2023, after 10 months of LDN therapy, she successfully stopped taking coxibs without any deterioration in her condition. At that point, her LDN dose was 4.5 mg. In January 2024, she reached her "happy dose," consisting of 1 mg in the morning and 4.5 mg in the evening, totalling 5.5 mg. She remarked that this morning dose was what she had been lacking. A higher dose of 6 mg was poorly tolerated.

In January 2024, a densitometry test was ordered. The DEXA test revealed the lowest T-Score of -2.2 in L2 (indicating advanced osteopenia). Additionally, the TBS (trabecular bone score) showed features of osteoporosis in the L1-L3 vertebrae (T-score -2.5). The L4 vertebra could not be considered in relation to the previous lumbar stabilization procedure. She began supplementing with calcium, and after six months, follow-up DEXA showed stabilization of the T-score, although there was a worsening in the TBS score for L1-L3, which measured -3.2. The next DEXA scan is planned for January 2025. During the upcoming check-up, it will be decided whether treatment with bisphosphonates or denosumab is necessary.

Expected Outcome
We expected the patient to feel better overall. We anticipated improvements in mobility, pain relief, and a lower risk of needing more aggressive treatments.

Actual Outcome
Thanks to the positive results from the LDN therapy, she feels very well and has reported no pain. She has not required more aggressive treatments that could potentially cause complications or adverse events. Currently, she can walk 7 km without deteriorating her condition. Furthermore, her rheumatology consultations are less frequent; the last one took place in August 2024.

Conclusion
A relatively new approach involving low-dose naltrexone (LDN) is not yet widely recognized among rheumatologists; however, some dermatologists are exploring its use in treating patients with psoriasis and PsA, both systematically and topically. Recently, initial publications have emerged in this area. (Weinstock LB, et al., 2020; Joanna Jaros and Peter Lio 2019).

Given the pleiotropic effects of LDN on chronic inflammation, it should be considered for cases of psoriasis and psoriatic arthritis. Continued research is necessary to promote understanding of LDN as an effective and cost-effective therapy. (Jarred Younger, Luke Parkitny, and David McLain 2014; Phillip S. Kim and Michael A. Fishman 2020; Jarred Younger et al., 2013; Karlo Toljan and Bruce Vrooman 2018).

LDN therapy should be considered a very effective approach for cases of psoriatic arthritis, especially when there is intense pain.

Symptom Relief for Rheumatoid Arthritis

Rachel Noonan, PharmD

Abstract

Early signs of inexplicable, debilitating pain in a teenage patient proved challenging when providers failed to believe her symptoms. Ultimately diagnosed with rheumatoid arthritis by the age of 13, JG juggled multiple therapies to keep flares at bay for over 20 years. The autoimmune disease continued to cause challenging bouts of inflammatory pain until late 2022, when she was introduced to low-dose naltrexone (LDN). In a case study that mirrors promising current research, initiating compounded LDN tablets and maintaining daily administration of 4.5 mg for over 3 years decreased JG's flare frequency and severity, improved symptomology, and reduced her medication burden.

Introduction

While targeted therapies can temporarily manage autoimmune disease-related pain, many patients tolerate limited quality of life and progressively decline. Rheumatoid arthritis (RA) is no different. A condition defined by inflammatory joint pain rife with unpredictable flares, RA often requires multiple therapeutic modalities to address symptom relief and disease progression.

In Raknes (et al.) retrospective review involving RA patients, persistent daily LDN administration at doses <5 mg was associated with a 13% daily dose reduction of all other medications (P<.003) after one year of intervention. The medications investigators found reduced in this analysis are typically paramount to comprehensive RA care, such as non-steroidal anti-inflammatories (NSAIDs), corticosteroids, opioids, disease-modifying antirheumatic drugs (DMARDs), and tumor necrosis factor-alpha inhibitors. Medication fill history of the 180 patients receiving persistent LDN therapy revealed LDN's potential ability to minimize chronic pain-related medication load in rheumatic conditions. (Raknes, Guttorm, and Lars Småbrekke 2019).

JG is a practicing healthcare professional and parent of two young children in her late 30s, who, despite years of targeted therapy, continued to experience crippling flares associated with rheumatoid arthritis.

Patient Description
- Age/Height/Weight: 37, 5'8", 142 lbs
- No tobacco use
- Alcohol 1-2 drinks 1-2 times per month
- Occasional caffeine
- Exercise 1-3 times per week (weightlifting and yoga)
- Allergies (Drugs): Levaquin (levofloxacin) – hallucinations
- Occupation: Registered Nurse, lactation consultant
- OTC Med History: Fish oil, Folic acid, Multivitamin, Probiotic, B-complex, Melatonin
- Medical Conditions and Diseases: Rheumatoid arthritis, depression and anxiety
- Current RX History: Bupropion 300 XR po daily, LDN 4.5 mg po daily, Adalimumab 40 mg subcutaneous weekly, Methotrexate 15 mg subcutaneous weekly
- Relevant Family Medical History: Mom diagnosed with fibromyalgia

History
Teen patient JG presents with inexplicable pain roughly two weeks after recovering from the flu in 2001. The discomfort began as bilateral pain in the toes and ankles, progressively moving up the body and spreading to the knees, hips, elbows, and wrists. Described

as intense, aching, deep-seated pain in the joints, it quickly became sharp, shooting pain with activity. Coupled with swelling and discoloration, particularly in the toes, knees, and fingers, within a few short weeks, JG found herself completely debilitated by the pain. She was only 13 years old and could not walk downstairs or lift a milk carton from the refrigerator.

After her primary care provider ran tests for Lyme disease that were negative, JG suffered six more months of troubling symptoms due to insufficient medical care. Unable to pinpoint a sufficient cause for JG's mysterious symptomology, her PCP went as far as to suggest she was fabricating her condition. She was prescribed high-dose prednisone for months on end, resulting in significant side effects such as moon face and lipomas, before the patient was finally referred to a rheumatologist.

Despite negative serum tests, which can be common in younger patient populations, JG's ANA and CRP were high enough to point to a proper diagnosis of rheumatoid arthritis. She started immunomodulatory agent leflunomide oral tablets at 20 mg daily and continued therapy for roughly 6 months without experiencing any real relief from the pain. The provider then converted JG to etanercept, injecting subcutaneously twice monthly, which helped to reduce her symptoms significantly, but not completely. Increasing etanercept frequency to once weekly administration finally proved successful, and JG felt genuine relief from her excruciating pain for the first time since symptom onset.

While etanercept was effective for nearly 10 years, it was not enough to keep flares entirely at bay. Oral prednisone bursts were necessary a few times every year, with the occasional injectable methylprednisolone required. Steroids caused JG significant side effects, preventing sleep. Within a couple of years of starting the recombinant DNA-derived protein, JG began to require weekly oral methotrexate administration to manage breakthrough flares, which eventually turned into weekly injections. When her flares became more frequent and more challenging to manage, JG transitioned etanercept therapy to certolizumab 200 mg every other week unsuccessfully for 2 months before starting adalimumab 40 mg subcutaneously weekly in 2012. Adalimumab and methotrexate weekly have been the mainstay of her RA treatment plan ever since.

Adalimumab and methotrexate have been a success for JG, but she still suffered from flares multiple times a year, often due to stress or illness. Managing unpredictable bouts of physical impairment continued to interrupt her daily life. It wasn't until she was introduced to LDN by a trusted friend and compounding pharmacist that her rheumatoid arthritis transformed into a condition she could successfully manage with confidence.

Treatment Plan
LDN 1 mg tablets by mouth daily, slowly increasing the dose by ½ tablets every week as tolerated until reaching the target dose of 4.5 mg daily.

Maintain LDN 4.5 mg by mouth daily in conjunction with weekly adalimumab and methotrexate therapy.

Expected Outcome
Despite JG's rheumatologist's refusal to prescribe LDN, stating he considered the compound an "ineffective money grab," JG's primary care physician was compelled by LDN's immune modulation research JG's pharmacist had shared. The patient initiated therapy without significant clinical expectations from her healthcare provider.

Actual Outcome
JG shares that starting LDN was life-changing. Now that her RA-associated flares are limited to those only caused by interruptions in therapy or illness, bursts of prednisone to manage symptoms are now

unnecessary. Her energy levels are noticeably higher, she experiences no underlying aches in her joints as she did before therapy, and she believes herself less prone to injury. "Before, I would go for a hike and experience pain in my knees for days afterward. Now, I have no residual inflammation or pain from strenuous activity."

Conclusion

Initiating daily LDN 4.5 mg as a complement to her existing RA drug regimen helped JG reduce the medications she once required to manage flares associated with her longstanding RA diagnosis. JG's improved symptomology and decreased flare frequency highlight a vulnerable population experiencing the incredible quality-of-life benefits with the addition of low-dose naltrexone. (Rupp, Adam et al., 2023).

Eosinophilic Granulomatosis with Polyangiitis

Edyta Biernat-Kaluza, MD, PhD

Abstract

A 64-year-old woman has been suffering from eosinophilic granulomatosis with polyangiitis (EGPA), formerly known as Churg-Strauss syndrome, for the past 19 years. Her diagnosis came after eight years of various signs and symptoms. Clinical manifestations included hypereosinophilia, a cough that was initially recognized as bronchial asthma but was later misdiagnosed as a tuberculosis infection. Additionally, she experienced severe sinusitis and neurological symptoms, such as peroneal nerve paresis and intense systemic pain.

Her condition improved with a few months of steroid and cyclophosphamide therapy. However, she later faced complications, including a fracture of the T11 vertebra, recurrent sinusitis, and pneumonia with pleuritis. Prior to modifying her therapy with low-dose naltrexone (LDN), mitoceuticals, vitamin D3, probiotics, butyric acid, and adrenal support, she was weak, had difficulty speaking, and suffered from frequent infections.

After adopting this holistic and partly complementary approach, her immune function, pain levels, general well-being, laboratory results, and quality of life have significantly improved. LDN therapy has been shown to be particularly effective for this type of vasculitis.

Introduction

Churg-Strauss syndrome, also known as eosinophilic granulomatosis with polyangiitis (EGPA), is a rare and severe form of vasculitis that affects small blood vessels and medium-sized arteries. This life-threatening rheumatological condition presents with a variety of interdisciplinary symptoms.

Pulmonary manifestations include asthma and transient infiltrates visible on radiographs. Hematological symptoms are characterized by hypereosinophilia, while neurological symptoms can result in mono- or polyneuropathy. Additionally, laryngological symptoms may involve abnormalities in the paranasal sinuses.

The main treatments for Churg-Strauss syndrome typically involve steroids combined with immunosuppressants. Cyclophosphamide was commonly used in the past, while rituximab, an anti-CD20 antibody targeting B lymphocytes, has been used more recently. Although steroids are effective in managing the condition, they can lead to well-known complications such as hypertension, infections, osteoporosis, and diabetes mellitus. As a result, it is important to consider adjunctive treatments or complementary approaches aimed at reducing the vasculitis damage index (VDI). (EULAR Textbook on the Rheumatic Diseases; Editor Johannes WJ Bijlsma; 2012; BMJ Group, Karlo Toljan and Bruce Vrooman 2018).

In a case involving a patient with Churg-Strauss syndrome, despite having received effective treatment with steroids and cyclophosphamide, the patient reported a significant improvement in her general condition and quality of life after undergoing low-dose naltrexone (LDN) therapy.

Patient Description

A 64-year-old woman appeared for the first time in my office in September 2023 with a primary diagnosis of Churg-Strauss syndrome (a type of vasculitis), also known as eosinophilic granulomatosis with polyangiitis (EGPA).

History

Her medical issues began in childhood, starting with skin psoriasis that disappeared during puberty. After completing her studies, she developed gallbladder stones. Instead of opting for surgery, she chose to dissolve them using lemon juice, which provided good, though not perfect, results; she still has one stone.

Later on, she experienced recurrent infections, particularly angina, and sinusitis with polyps, which required numerous rounds of antibiotics. In 2006, at the age of 44, she developed a chronic cough for the first time, accompanied by hypereosinophilia at 20%. The cough was very productive despite her not being a smoker. She was ultimately diagnosed with bronchial asthma, and tropical eosinophilia was ruled out due to her many trips to China between 2000 and 2008.

By the end of 2009, her worsening cough led to a misdiagnosis of a tuberculosis (TB) infection, and she underwent a month of anti-*Mycobacterium* treatment. During this treatment, she developed neurological issues, including paresis of the left peroneal nerve. After extensive neurological diagnostics, she received a diagnosis of axonal neuropathy. Myositis was ruled out, but there remained an unresolved suspicion of muscular dystrophy.

After seven years of various examinations, in the end, she was diagnosed in 2013 with Churg-Strauss syndrome, characterized by bronchial asthma, nasal polyps, sinusitis, heart involvement, hypereosinophilia, and positive former anti-perinuclear cytoplasmic antibodies p-ANCA, despite currently testing negative for both: anti-perinuclear cytoplasmic antibodies p-ANCA and antineutrophil cytoplasmic antibodies (c-ANCA). She underwent treatment with systemic steroids and cyclophosphamide for eight months, which yielded good results.

In 2014, she was diagnosed with a pulmonary embolism due to the Factor V Leiden mutation, and in 2015, she began taking rivaroxaban at a dosage of 20 mg. She also suffered a fracture of the T11 vertebra, for which she received oral bisphosphonate therapy (ibandronic acid, administered once a month).

Her family has a history of neurological issues; her sister suffers from muscular dystrophy, and spasticity is also present in the family. Both her father and sister have been diagnosed with lung embolisms. When she noticed new neurological symptoms, such as tingling, she modified her diet by eliminating certain foods, particularly cruciferous vegetables and most grains, although she occasionally eats rice. Her diet is high in animal proteins, resembling a paleo diet. Concurrently, she began using natural supplements like vilcacora, cordyceps fungi, and maca, providing good results.

In 2019, she was diagnosed with another autoimmune condition: Graves' disease, for which she was treated with thiamazole for one year and underwent iodotherapy twice. In 2022, she experienced pneumonia with pleuritis. Currently, she is awaiting admission to an endocrinology clinic.

Physical Examination

When I met her for the first time in September 2023, she appeared very thin and cachectic, exhibiting a deep, productive cough. Due to her dyspnea, she spoke with difficulty. Throughout the consultation, the patient frequently cleared her throat. Her body weight was 48.5 kg, her height was 164 cm, and her BMI was 18.03.

The rheumatological examination revealed atrophy of the temporal and masseter muscles and atrophy of the quadriceps muscle in her thigh. Additionally, there were weakened reflexes in the left foot and tenderness in both metatarsal joints, especially on the left side. Furthermore, she reported systemic pain rated 7 out of 10 on the Visual Analog Scale (VAS).

Test Results

Summary of Important Hospital Tests 2009:

- Eosinophilia: 57% (normal <6%)
- CPK: 581 (normal range: 26–140)

- D-dimers: 1209 (normal <500)
- ANA: Negative
- LKM: Negative
- AMA: Negative
- p-ANCA: Positive at a ratio of 1:1280
- ANCA: Negative
- Chest CT: Ground-glass changes observed in the upper part of both lungs
- EMG: suggested the presence of myotonic dystrophy and severe axonal neuropathy
- MRI of lumbar region: Dehydration of L4-L5 and L5-S1 discs

Summary of Important Hospital Tests 2013:
- Eosinophilia: 17.2% (normal <6%)
- ANCA: Negative
- c-ANCA: Negative
- Bronchoscopy with BAL: Normal number of eosinophils
- CT of sinuses: Massive inflammatory changes with occlusion of ductal complexes
- MRI of the heart: Shows active inflammation that is typical for hypereosinophilia, involving the subendocardial layers

First Visit at Rheumatological Outpatient Clinic (September 2023):
- Eosinophilia: 10.6% (normal <6%)
- Hypoalbuminemia: 49.7% - 3.63 g/dl (normal range: 4.02-4.76)
- DHEAS: 7.7 µg/dl (normal range: 29.7-260)

Latest Results at Rheumatological Outpatient Clinic (January 2025):
- Eosinophilia: 9.3% (normal <6%)
- Albumin levels: 61.7% - 4.2 g/dl (normal range: 4.02-4.76)
- DHEAS: 185 µg/dl (normal range: 29.7-260)

Diagnoses:
- Churg-Strauss syndrome (eosinophilic granulomatosis with polyangiitis, EGPA)
- Bronchial asthma
- Axonal neuropathy
- Skin psoriasis
- Graves' disease
- Osteoporosis with Th11 fracture
- Gallstones

Treatment Plan and Outcome

After I recommended low-dose naltrexone (LDN), she chose to begin this new treatment. The initial dose of LDN was 0.25 mg, which was to be increased by 0.5 mg every ten days until reaching 1.5 mg. She expressed a desire to use higher doses as soon as possible, so we agreed to raise the LDN dose by 0.5 mg every ten days. After six weeks of using LDN, she reported feeling increased energy, improved mobility, and less pain in both feet. Her current dose is now 6 mg, and we are still working to find her "happy dose." She is very optimistic and wishes to be treated with the highest possible dose.

In addition to LDN, she has been following other complementary holistic treatments, including vitamin D3 in the form of calcifediol, probiotics, and mitoceutics such as CoQ10, alpha-lipoic acid, and NAC, along with butyric acid. We used the plant version (Catalpa/Surmia) to support her adrenal health and later introduced a chemical (DHEA). She has also been taking Ecomer (shark liver oil) and vitamin B6.

Her immune system has improved significantly, and she firmly believes that her current condition results from the LDN treatment. Due to osteoporosis with a vertebral fracture of Th11 (postmenopausal, after steroid treatment, and possibly as a result of anticoagulant therapy with rivaroxaban), I proposed modifying her bisphosphonate treatment. Instead of oral ibandronate, we decided to switch to intravenous zoledronic acid (5 mg), and she received her first dose in February 2024. A follow-up bone density scan, including TBS (trabecular bone score), is planned for February 2025, after which she may receive the next dose of intravenous zoledronic acid.

Not only has her clinical condition improved, especially her cough, but she also reported reduced systemic pain (her VAS score decreased from 7/10 to 2/10). Her laboratory tests showed improvements, with elevated LDH, hypoalbuminemia, and reduced DHEA levels all corrected.

She visited my office for the last time in January 2025 and presented much better. She gained a few kilograms, bringing her current weight to 50 kg, with a BMI of 18.6. Her cough has become rare, her breathing is easier, and her nose is less congested. She can talk without any difficulties.

She is delighted with the LDN therapy and has signed an informed consent to use her medical data anonymously to help promote LDN as a treatment option for rare conditions, such as Churg-Strauss syndrome (EGPA). To the best of my knowledge, this is the first report in the medical literature about using LDN as an option for complementary therapy in Churg-Strauss syndrome (EGPA).

Conclusion
LDN therapy should be considered an effective approach for vasculitis, particularly when systemic pain is present. (Jarred Younger, Luke Parkitny, and David McLain 2014; Norman Brown, Jaak Panksepp 2009; Jarred Younger et al., 2013; Phillip S. Kim and Michael A. Fishman 2020).

Managing Refractory Symptoms in Crohn's Disease

Scott Mortenson, MD

Abstract

A 35-year-old male with Crohn's disease presented with persistent abdominal pain and inflammatory markers despite being on a stable regimen of adalimumab. Low-dose naltrexone (LDN) at 4.5 mg nightly was introduced alongside targeted peptide therapy to enhance gut barrier integrity and modulate immune function. After 8 weeks, the patient reported a 60% reduction in abdominal pain, decreased bowel urgency, and improved energy levels. CRP levels dropped from 25 mg/L to 8 mg/L, and fecal calprotectin was reduced by 50%. This case underscores LDN's potential role as an adjunct in Crohn's disease management, particularly in patients with refractory symptoms.

Introduction

Crohn's disease is a chronic inflammatory bowel disorder characterized by persistent gastrointestinal inflammation, abdominal pain, diarrhea, and systemic symptoms such as fatigue and weight loss. Standard treatment strategies include biologics (e.g., TNF inhibitors like adalimumab), corticosteroids, and immunosuppressants, yet many patients continue to experience breakthrough symptoms.

LDN, a partial opioid receptor antagonist, has demonstrated promising results in autoimmune conditions by modulating glial cell activation, T-cell function, and pro-inflammatory cytokines (PMC, 2022). Additionally, emerging research highlights the role of peptides such as BPC-157, KPV, and thymosin alpha-1 in promoting gut healing and immune balance. This case report explores how LDN, combined with peptide therapy, successfully reduced inflammation and symptom severity in a patient with treatment-resistant Crohn's disease.

Patient Description
A 35-year-old Hispanic male, single, working as a graphic designer, with an 8-year history of Crohn's disease. He led a sedentary lifestyle, had previously been on corticosteroids, and had failed multiple dietary interventions before resorting to biologic therapy.

History
The patient was diagnosed with Crohn's disease at age 27 after experiencing chronic diarrhea, weight loss, and severe abdominal pain. He was placed on adalimumab (40 mg subcutaneously every two weeks) but continued to struggle with persistent abdominal pain (5/10), occasional diarrhea (3-5 episodes per week), and fatigue. He had been steroid-dependent in the past but was eager to explore additional interventions to reduce his reliance on immunosuppressive medications.

Physical and Psychiatric Examination Results
- General appearance: No acute distress
- Abdomen: Mild tenderness in the right lower quadrant, no peritoneal signs
- Neurological and psychiatric: Normal cognition, mild reactive anxiety related to chronic illness

Laboratory and Imaging Results:
- CRP: 25 mg/L (elevated, indicative of ongoing inflammation)
- Fecal Calprotectin: 300 µg/g (suggestive of active disease)
- Vitamin D: 22 ng/mL (low)
- Zonulin: Elevated (suggesting increased intestinal permeability)

- Microbiome Analysis: Decreased Akkermansia and Faecalibacterium prausnitzii (markers of dysbiosis and gut inflammation)

Treatment Plan

Given his ongoing symptoms despite biologic therapy, the following adjunctive treatments were introduced:

Immune Modulation and Inflammation Control:

- Low-dose naltrexone (LDN) 1.5 mg titrated to 4.5 mg nightly – Downregulates inflammation, reduces intestinal permeability and promotes Treg cell function.
- Thymosin Alpha-1 (TA1) – 1.5 mg subcutaneous (SC) 2x/ week – Enhances immune balance, reduces autoimmunity, and boosts mucosal immunity.

Gut Repair and Mucosal Healing:

- BPC-157 – 500 mcg SC daily – Accelerates healing of intestinal epithelial cells, reduces gut permeability, and promotes angiogenesis in damaged tissue.
- KPV – 500 mcg SC or oral spray daily – Anti-inflammatory tripeptide that modulates mast cell activity and reduces histamine-related gut symptoms.
- Plaquex IV (Phosphatidylcholine 50 mg 2x/week) – Strengthens cellular membranes, reduces oxidative stress, and supports bile flow for improved digestion.
- Gut Feeling Supplement (BPC-157 + KPV + Akkermansia + Immunolin®) – 1 scoop daily – Supports microbiome diversity and intestinal lining integrity.

Mitochondrial and Systemic Support:
- NAD+ IV (200 mg 1-2x/week) + MOTS-c (5 mg SC 3x/week) + SS-31 (5 mg SC daily) – Enhances mitochondrial function and energy production to counteract Crohn's-related fatigue.
- Vitamin D3/K2 (5,000 IU daily) – Addresses deficiency and modulates immune responses.

Expected Outcome
- Reduction in abdominal pain by 40% within 8 weeks.
- Improved stool consistency and reduced diarrhea frequency.
- CRP decrease to <10 mg/L as inflammation resolves.
- Improved energy levels with mitochondrial support.

Actual Outcome
At 8 weeks, the patient reported:
- Pain decreased from 5/10 to 2/10 (60% improvement).
- Bowel movements normalized to 1-2 formed stools per day (no diarrhea).
- Fatigue improved significantly, allowing him to work full-time without midday crashes.
- CRP dropped to 8 mg/L, indicating lower systemic inflammation.
- Fecal calprotectin decreased to 120 µg/g, suggesting improved gut integrity.

He tolerated LDN well with no significant side effects, aside from mild insomnia during the first two weeks, which resolved spontaneously.

Conclusion
This case highlights LDN's role as an adjunctive therapy in Crohn's disease, particularly for patients who remain symptomatic

despite biologics. By modulating immune activity and reducing neuroinflammation, LDN contributed to significant symptom relief. Additionally, targeted peptides (BPC-157, KPV, TA1) accelerated gut healing, reduced intestinal permeability, and restored microbiome balance.

For clinicians treating Crohn's, this case supports:

- LDN as a valuable adjunct for inflammatory pain management.
- Peptides (BPC-157, KPV) as key tools in gut repair.
- Mitochondrial support (NAD+, MOTS-c, SS-31) to counteract Crohn's-related fatigue.

Future studies should further explore LDN's impact on gut permeability, microbiome restoration, and long-term remission rates in inflammatory bowel disease.

Overcoming Juvenile Dermatomyositis

Sebastian Denison, RPh

Abstract

LDN is currently understood to have impacts on patients who have significant immune dysfunction that causes serious health problems along a continuum that generally leads to autoimmune disorders. Many of these patients suffer from multiple symptoms, including mobility dysfunction, muscle weakness, and different pain scenarios. Many autoimmune patients complain of pain in joints and muscles, as well as nerve pain and, finally, headaches. Pain is subjective, but when a patient describes pain, it is personal and changes not just the patient's life but those around the patient.

When the patient is young and facing a lifetime of pain, the parents become advocates to healthcare providers who may not fully understand the depth of the problem. In many cases, the parents might be a health care provider themselves and ask, 'Is there more we can do?" and in this case, that's precisely what occurred.

Introduction

The patient was 5 years old (m) when his mother first noticed he was having rashes around his eyes and joint pain. This was initially thought of as mild eczema, but the pain persisted, and he started showing signs of muscle weakness and chronic fatigue. Eventually, as the parents persisted that the treatments were not improving his condition, he was referred to a pediatrician who was able to diagnose the patient with Juvenile Dermatomyositis (JDM). (Gara, Soumaya et al., 2023)

This rare inflammatory autoimmune disease primarily affects children, causing inflammation of the muscles, calcium deposits, skin rashes, and pain. Long-term consequences for these patients, left untreated, are muscle weakness, gastrointestinal vascular inflammation, cardiovascular complications, heart failure, and breathing problems. Finally, the calcium deposits in the skin and muscles leave bumps and are intensely painful.

Patient Description
The patient was a five-year-old boy when the health problems began.

History
When he was finally diagnosed, he needed assistance to roll over in bed, frequent rests when playing, and help getting up off the ground. His initial treatment was the common standard of care with both methotrexate and corticosteroids, and the patient was monitored for changes in liver enzymes to ensure that he was not inappropriately dosed.

After a few years, the patient was again struggling and was not gaining weight or muscle mass as normal kids do. He was still experiencing pain and problems, and his liver enzymes started to climb. He was initiated on Intravenous Immunoglobulin (IVIG) therapy. (Arumugham, Vijay B., and Appaji Rayi. 2023). This is done in many patients with autoimmune disorders to help fight infection and mitigate some of the autoimmune effects. The rheumatologist also recommended adding mycophenolate (a potent immunosuppressant drug) or exploring biological therapy (antibodies that target inflammatory cytokines) as an option. Biologics in pediatrics are now more commonly used but still have not fully been explored as a treatment option in this patient group and come with their own set of side effects.

IGIV therapy and Biologic therapy differ as one gives components of the immune system designed to support good immune function, whereas the biologics give components to target inflammatory cytokines that limit inflammation but also compromise adaptive immune function. This is where the pharmacist mother started asking questions about LDN for her son.

Treatment Plan
The team had some questions and initially was resistant to the addition of LDN to his therapy, but the primary care physician prescribed it at a dose of 0.5 mg daily.

Expected Outcome
The intent was to minimize the inflammation and rash, improve mobility and energy, and decrease overall pain perception.

Actual Outcome
Two months later, his dose was increased to 1 mg daily as improvement had been noted. Within another 6 months (as he grew), the dose was increased to 2 mg daily with 0.5 mg increments, with continued improvement.

This was an update from his mother;

His calcium deposits (which we were told would never resolve once they appeared) have all gone. As far as muscle disease, he has no aches or weakness. He got a perfect score on the childhood myositis assessment score (which the physiotherapist said he's never seen in this disease before). He has never had a perfect score in the past. His high sensitivity C-reactive protein (inflammatory marker) has been consistently unmeasurable at less than 0.3. He plays baseball, tackle football, and any sport he can manage to get involved in without any issues; in fact, he is usually the team's star.

In November 2020, he was told he had no evidence of disease with respect to labs, visual exam, or physio exam. He has not experienced any notable side effects from LDN throughout the entire time, including initiation.

In January of 2025, he continued to be a perfectly normal, healthy, active, pain-free teenager with no signs of disease, and the only medication at the time of writing was the LDN.

Conclusion

What was very interesting was that not only did his pain and other symptoms improve, but he started to grow and thrive like other kids his age. He gained muscle mass, improved height and weight, improved in activities, and had more energy every day.

At the same time, the team was able to decrease and eventually discontinue the methotrexate entirely, with liver function fully returning to normal. His dose was slowly titrated as he grew based on need, and he is fully stable at 3 mg. His pain has entirely resolved, there are no restrictions on activities, and every time I speak with his mother, there is good news.

Acknowledgement: The pharmacy team at Irsfeld Pharmacy in Dickerson, ND, provided the data for this case study using their online symptom tracking system, which they developed.

Immune Dysregulation and Neurological Symptoms

Scott Mortenson, MD

Abstract

This case study examines the impact of low-dose naltrexone (LDN) on a 42-year-old female with a past medical history of polycystic ovary syndrome (PCOS) who was suffering from chronic immune dysregulation, neuroinflammation, and persistent neurological symptoms following a tick-borne Babesia infection and environmental toxin exposure.

The patient presented with severe fatigue, cognitive impairment, autonomic instability, and clotting abnormalities, all of which worsened after prolonged mold exposure. Standard treatments, including antimicrobials, detoxification therapies, and immune modulators, provided only temporary relief.

This case demonstrates how LDN was successfully integrated into a comprehensive treatment plan, significantly improving neurological function, immune stability, and overall systemic inflammation.

Introduction

Tick-borne infections such as Babesia, particularly in combination with mold exposure and chronic inflammatory syndromes, create a unique challenge for both diagnosis and treatment. Patients often present with fatigue, clotting abnormalities, cognitive dysfunction, and persistent immune activation, yet conventional treatments targeting singular aspects of the illness frequently fail.

LDN has been recognized for its ability to modulate immune function, suppress excessive inflammatory responses, and improve neurological recovery by acting on opioid receptors and microglial regulation. This case illustrates how LDN was integrated into a broader systems-based approach to successfully reduce inflammation, regulate clotting, and restore energy production in a patient with treatment-resistant Babesia infection and immune dysfunction.

Patient Description

A 42-year-old female with a past medical history of PCOS presented with progressive neurological and systemic symptoms following a tick-borne infection and environmental mold exposure. Her primary complaints included chronic fatigue, cognitive fog, postural instability, and excessive clotting tendencies. She also experienced environmental sensitivities, food intolerances, and fluctuations in immune function.

History

Her symptoms initially began in her early thirties, worsening significantly after a prolonged undiagnosed tick bite and exposure to a mold-contaminated home. She developed increasing fatigue, autonomic dysfunction, cognitive decline, and a history of unexplained clotting events. Despite multiple medical evaluations, she was misdiagnosed with anxiety, depression, and functional neurological disorders.

After several failed treatments—including standard Babesia protocols, detox regimens, and immune therapies—her condition remained refractory. Seeking a more comprehensive approach, she underwent advanced testing, which revealed persistent Babesia infection, immune dysregulation, and clotting dysfunction.

Physical and Neurological Examination Results

- Cognitive Dysfunction: Severe brain fog, slow processing speed, and difficulty concentrating.
- Immune Dysregulation: Chronic inflammation, histamine intolerance, and suspected mast cell activation.

- Neurological Findings: Sensory hypersensitivity, postural dizziness, and mild tremors.
- Clotting Dysfunction: History of micro-clots and sluggish circulation.
- Autonomic Dysregulation: Fluctuating blood pressure, temperature intolerance, and tachycardia.

Test Results
Babesia Testing:
- Babesia duncani (WA1) IgG: 1:256 – Highly elevated, suggesting chronic or active Babesia infection.

Coagulation and Clotting Markers:
- Fibrin Monomer: Elevated – Suggesting hypercoagulability and excessive fibrin formation.
- Thrombin-Antithrombin (TAT) Complex: 4.5 pmol/L – Increased thrombin activity indicating a clotting disorder.

Mycotoxin Panel:
- Elevated Gliotoxin and Cladosporium herbarum IgG – confirming persistent mold exposure.

Immune Dysfunction:
- Eosinophil Cationic Protein (ECP): 14 ng/mL – Indicating chronic immune activation.
- Thyroid Peroxidase (TPO) Antibodies: 65 IU/mL – Suggesting autoimmune thyroid involvement.

Metabolic Dysfunction:
- Low CO_2 (18 mmol/L) – Suggesting mild metabolic acidosis, often linked to chronic inflammation and mitochondrial dysfunction.

Treatment Plan

Given the severity of immune dysfunction, neurological impairment, and clotting abnormalities, the treatment plan prioritized immune stabilization and mitochondrial recovery before antimicrobial therapy and detoxification.

Primary Interventions:

- T3 (5 mcg BID, adjusted as needed) – Supports mitochondrial function and metabolic balance.
- Tirzepatide 1.75 mg a week titrated to 2.5 mg for insulin, weight, and PCOS control.
- Plaquex IV (Phosphatidylcholine 50 mg 2x/week) – Enhances cell membrane integrity, clotting regulation, and toxin clearance.

Immune and Clotting Regulation: Low-dose naltrexone (LDN):

- Started at 1.5 mg nightly, titrated to 4.5 mg over six weeks.
- Goal: Modulates immune function, reduces neuroinflammation, and stabilizes clotting.

Gut and Mast Cell Regulation:

- Gut Feeling Supplement – BPC-157 (500 mcg), KPV (250 mcg), Akkermansia, Immunolin to restore gut integrity.
- Thymosin Alpha-1 (1.5 mg 2x/week) + LL-37 (200 mcg daily) – Targets chronic infections and supports immune function.

Biofilm Disruption and Babesia Eradication:

- Lumbrokinase (50 mg daily) + Nattokinase (100 mg daily) – Dissolves fibrin-related biofilms and improves circulation.
- BEG Nasal Spray (2x daily) + Xylitol Nasal Spray (2x daily) – Clears nasal biofilm reservoirs.
- EBOO IV (weekly, four sessions) – Facilitates mycotoxin and pathogen clearance.

Mitochondrial and Neuroimmune Support:

- NAD+ IV (1-2x/week) + MOTS-c (5 mg 3x/week) + SS-31 (5 mg daily subQ) – Repairs mitochondrial damage and reverses neuroinflammation.
- Cerebropep / Cerebrolysin: Enhances neuroplasticity and cognitive function.

Expected Outcome

The patient was expected to experience:

- Reduction in neuroinflammation and cognitive dysfunction (via LDN, Semax, and detox support).
- Stabilization of mast cell reactivity and clotting abnormalities.
- Improved mitochondrial function and energy production.
- Reduction in Babesia burden and systemic immune activation.

Actual Outcome

After eight weeks of therapy, including LDN titration, mitochondrial repair, and immune stabilization, the patient reported substantial improvements:

- Brain fog improved from 9/10 severity to 2/10.
- Sustained energy levels improved by 80%.
- Clotting symptoms reduced significantly.
- MCAS-related sensitivities markedly decreased.

The patient experienced further cognitive and immune gains by twelve weeks, with improved temperature regulation and reduced clotting risk. LDN played a pivotal role in regulating the immune response and supporting mitochondrial function, allowing other therapies to be more effective.

Conclusion

This case highlights LDN's role as a critical immunomodulator in chronic Babesia infections. LDN was a key therapy in turning a previously refractory case into a successful recovery trajectory by reducing neuroinflammation, stabilizing clotting pathways, and improving mitochondrial function.

Key Takeaways for Practitioners:

- LDN is highly effective when used alongside mitochondrial and clotting support.
- Slow titration (1.5 mg → 4.5 mg over six weeks) prevents excessive immune activation.
- LDN should be included in tick-borne disease treatment when neuroinflammation and clotting dysfunction are present.

This patient achieved measurable, sustainable improvements by integrating LDN into a broader systems-based approach, reinforcing its importance in treating Babesia, immune dysregulation, and neuroinflammatory conditions.

Pediatric Rheumatoid Arthritis without DMARDS

Paul S. Anderson, NMD

Abstract

A thirteen-year-old female presented to our clinic at the referral of her primary care physician. She was diagnosed with pediatric rheumatoid arthritis at the age of ten.

Between the ages of ten and thirteen, her pain and joint dysfunction progressed, and she was prescribed methotrexate.

She presented to the clinic with her parents with the goal of decreasing and, if possible, discontinuing her methotrexate.

Introduction

A thirteen-year-old female and her parents presented to the clinic upon the referral of her primary care physician. She had been diagnosed with juvenile rheumatoid arthritis at the age of ten following a number of years of nondescript complaints of joint pain. She was currently under the care of a pediatric rheumatologist and her primary care physician.

Between the ages of ten and thirteen, she had developed classic radiographic signs of rheumatic changes in the right wrist and left ankle. Her laboratory tests were normal with the exception of an elevated rheumatoid factor. She was placed on methotrexate as well as PRN NSAID medications. She and her parents expressed a desire to modify the disease without staying on methotrexate.

I collaborated with her primary care physician to obtain additional laboratory studies and explained to the family, patient, primary care physician, and rheumatologist that if we could assess comorbid conditions and treat them (as well as adding nutrient support and possibly low-dose naltrexone) we could potentially reduce or discontinue the methotrexate.

All parties agreed to the plan, and the rheumatologist agreed to monitor her disease and decrease or discontinue the methotrexate when appropriate.

Patient Presented with the Following Complaints
- Fatigue
- Pain in the rheumatic joints with any exercise
- Swelling in the rheumatic joints with any exercise

Test Results

Assessment of comorbidity / other health conditions based on new lab tests included:
- Low Vitamin D
- Low Vitamin B12
- Mild Hypothyroid state
- Positive food allergens
- Dietary imbalance – low protein intake with high carbohydrate intake

Treatment Plan
- Begin treating the above co-morbid conditions with Thyroid Rx., Vitamin D, a multi-vitamin with active forms of the B complex vitamins. She also initiated an Omega-3 supplement taken once daily with food.
- Begin to modify her diet to eliminate food allergens and increase protein intake while reducing simple carbohydrate intake. Increase hydration throughout the day.
- Began using a chart to monitor her energy, pain, and joint swelling.
- Initiated an oral low-dose naltrexone (LDN) taper based on her body weight. An adult dose equivalent of 4.5 mg is 0.065 mg/kg of body weight. This body weight-adjusted dose was

used as the goal dose. As a test dose, she started on half that dose for two weeks. After two weeks, she tolerated this test dose well and was raised to the full dose.

- Prior medications (methotrexate and NSAIDS) were maintained as previously prescribed.

Case Progression

We initially worked with her and the family regarding the implementation of the above plan. She had questions about the diet changes which we answered, and she was able to incorporate them with adequate compliance. She obtained all the prescriptions and supplements and began taking them immediately.

Over the course of the first three months, she expended most of her energy on making the necessary changes to her diet, as well as establishing a regular routine with her medication and supplement intake. Her pain, fatigue and joint swelling were not noticeably changed.

Between month four and month six she reported improved energy and sleep quality. She reported that the biggest aggravating activity for her joints was physical education (PE) class at school which she had an accommodation for (allowing her to stop activity if pain increased). A definite pattern of increased swelling and pain in the affected joints was observed following PE class activities. Because her energy and sleep were improved, it was easier for her to be more specific regarding the joint pain and swelling. She reported at the month six follow-up that she thought she might have experienced some reduction in pain and swelling after PE class, but it was subtle.

We followed her monthly between months six and twelve. Between months six and nine, her use of as-needed NSAIDS decreased greatly. Her fatigue and sleep improved and became more stable. Her pain and swelling from her PE class were also decreased. Based on this progress, we spoke to the rheumatologist, and she agreed that a methotrexate taper would be warranted. She had prior x-rays of the two affected joints from one and two years prior, which showed increased rheumatic degeneration at the second x-ray study. We ordered interval x-ray studies at the month eight visit to establish a baseline for monitoring potential progress and assessing the effect of the methotrexate decrease. The x-ray studies of the two affected joints showed no significant increase in rheumatic joint changes.

At month nine of our care plan, the rheumatologist started a tapered decrease in the methotrexate, which was planned for months nine through twelve. If she had any increase in pain or swelling that lasted more than a week, we would reconsider the methotrexate taper. One year into the plan of care, she was completely off the methotrexate, and she rarely needed the NSAIDS for pain.

Between the twelfth month of our care plan and the twenty-fourth month, we monitored her fatigue, sleep, swelling, pain, and her ability to maintain compliance with all the facets of the treatment plan. She tolerated the LDN well and the dose was stable throughout.

On the twenty-fourth month of our care plan, X-rays of the affected joints were ordered again. The rheumatologist agreed there was no interval worsening of her rheumatic joint changes. Her fatigue was mostly resolved. She rarely would have joint swelling following her exercise bouts, and her pain remained at very low levels.

Conclusion

She remains on the LDN, modified diet, and basic nutrients as her primary interventions. She has not had to return to using methotrexate or any other disease-modifying drugs for her rheumatoid arthritis.

Lyme Disease and Coinfections

Sarah J. Zielsdorf, MD, MS

Abstract

This is a case of a 56-year-old female with a history of multiple coinfections, autoimmunity, and chronic body pain, myalgias, fevers, migratory joint swelling, fatigue, brain fog, anemia, and elevated biomarkers indicating chronic inflammation. Low-dose naltrexone (LDN), in addition to other dietary and lifestyle modifications and therapeutic interventions, significantly helped the patient's quality of life via subjective improvements in pain and sleep and has been taken for more than eight years with sustained benefit. She has also had significant improvements in her labs, showing a persistent reduction in her chronic inflammatory markers.

Introduction

A hallmark of tick-borne and other co-infections is unchecked chronic inflammation, often with chronic downstream effects leading to post-treatment Lyme disease (PTLD). In 2012, clinician-researcher Richard Horowitz published a multifactorial model entitled Multiple Systemic Infectious Disease Syndrome (MSIDS), which identifies up to 16 overlapping sources of inflammation and their downstream effects. These categories must be individually evaluated and taken into account for patients to recover, and include infections, immune dysfunction/autoimmunity, inflammation, toxicity, allergies, nutritional and enzyme deficiencies, mitochondrial dysfunction, psychological dysfunction, neurological dysfunction, endocrine abnormalities, sleep disorders, autonomic nervous system dysfunction, gastrointestinal dysfunction, elevated liver enzymes, pain syndromes, and deconditioning. (Horowitz, Richard I. and Phyllis R. Freeman. 2018).

Lyme disease is known as the "great imitator" for myriad pain syndromes in every body system. The causative agent(s) induce systemic inflammation via the stimulation of chronic pro-inflammatory cytokine production (cell signals), including interleukin-1 (IL-1), IL-6, and tumor necrosis factor–alpha (TNF-α), which damage cell membranes, mitochondria, and nerve cells. Autoimmunity can happen if antibodies cross-react with tissue antigens. LDN is used off-label for the management of chronic infections of many types, including but not limited to viral, bacterial, fungal/yeast, and parasitic etiologies, as it reduces the chronic overproduction of pro-inflammatory cytokines. In Horowitz's open-label study of 500 patients with Lyme disease and MSIDS, approximately 75% of patients experienced less fatigue, joint, and muscle pain when the naltrexone dose was titrated to 4.5 mg at bedtime. (Alexander, Walter. 2012). In our experience, the dosing strategy for pain and inflammation may need to be higher in patients with malabsorptive conditions or split dosed.

Patient Description
A 56-year-old female with a past medical history significant for multiple tick-borne and viral infections vs rheumatoid arthritis-induced polyarthritis presented to our clinic with complaints of fatigue, muscle spasms, migraines, body pain and stiffness, with chronic migratory joint pain and swelling.

History
The patient described a history of multiple known tick bites and exposures from living in Illinois and visiting the East Coast, and previously tested positive for *Borrelia burgdorferi* antibodies (causative bacterial spirochete of Lyme disease), and given antimicrobial treatments (standard antibiotic course). The patient initially presented for total body pain and severe muscle spasms

in 2014 after a year of extreme stress and recurrent trauma, including a chronically abusive spouse and a new job as a caregiver for the elderly.

Her symptoms progressed until she required the use of a wheelchair for prolonged standing or ambulation. In 2017, on presentation to our clinic, her quality of life had diminished further, and she also endorsed recurrent chronic fevers with myalgias, severe brain fog, and depression. She rated her pain as unrelenting and 10/10 in intensity.

Physical Examination Results
Significant physical findings in 2017 included pain and swelling of multiple large and small joints, including knees, hips, wrists, and scattered MCP (metacarpophalangeal) and PIP (proximal interphalangeal) joints of her fingers. The patient ambulated with difficulty, muscles were diffusely tender to palpation, and several muscles were spastic. There were no focal neurological deficits.

Test Results
Initial labs in 2017 revealed significant and chronic fluctuating levels of hs-CRP (high sensitive C-Reactive Protein) of greater than 10 mg/L (elevated is greater than 3), ESR (Erythrocyte Sedimentation Rate) of 40mm/h, creatinine kinase with intermittently mild elevation, borderline low C4 and normal C3 complement proteins, elevated total complement, iron deficiency (microcytic)/inflammatory anemia (hemoglobin 9.0g/dL, normal range for an adult female 11.7-15.5g/dL), mildly positive Antinuclear Antibody (ANA) titer of 1:80, and elevated ferritin (acute phase reactant) of 450ng/mL (normal 16-288) with elevated platelet count upwards of 700,000/uL (normal upper limit is 400,000/uL).

Treatment Plan

A thorough workup of the patient was performed using a variety of autoimmunity and immune dysfunction, infectious disease serology, and direct testing methods. Additional antimicrobial therapies were used, though differentially tolerated. The patient maintained an intensive regimen of lifestyle modifications, including an anti-inflammatory elimination diet and stress mitigation and reduction of sympathetic nervous system dominance via vagal nerve stimulation exercises. Shortly after establishing care, the patient was initiated on LDN 1.5 mg but poorly tolerated aggressive titration and reduced to 0.375 mg nightly. With continued slow titration, she tolerated 4.5 mg by May of 2018. Of note, in 2018, her primary care physician changed her treatment regimen and included a homeopathic anti-inflammatory remedy, which induced a flare of her pain syndrome as well as ESR levels greater than 120mm/h (from baseline 40s). Her LDN dose was increased to 6 mg/nightly, which resolved the flare symptoms and calmed her inflammatory biomarkers with persistent resolution since that time.

Expected Outcome

The expected treatment outcome is improved quality of life with reduced inflammation on low-dose naltrexone and control of underlying chronic infections.

Actual Outcome

The patient no longer requires mobility assistance of any kind. She is able to exercise and play with her grandchildren. Her quality of life is excellent with controlled symptoms, including low pain levels, reduced joint swelling, and no muscle inflammation. Muscle spasms are rare. Fatigue is improved overall. The only major remaining symptom is waxing and waning brain fog. Her laboratory biomarkers have markedly improved, including a negative ANA, negative RF/CCP (Rheumatoid Factor and Cyclic Citrullinated Peptide) antibodies for rheumatoid arthritis, resolved ESR (average is now between 2-6mm/h), and hs-CRP (average is now 1.0 mg/L). With reduced inflammation, anemia was resolved (hemoglobin now 13.5g/dL), and ferritin and reactive thrombocytosis (elevated platelets) normalized.

Conclusion

LDN is an integral part of chronic illness management for the pleotropic effects on cells and impacts on both systemic unchecked inflammation and dysregulated immune responses. In this case, the patient's Lyme/RA arthritis imparts a high risk of coronary artery disease (CAD) – the impressive reduction of inflammatory biomarkers proves not only beneficial for this patient's quality of life but gives hope for her reduced cardiovascular risk and overall improved mortality benefit. One important recommendation for the use of LDN for Lyme and coinfections is to titrate LDN low and slow. The immune system is often "waking up" for the first time in potentially years, leading to potential strong side effects and initial intolerance of LDN, which simply means that the patient may have an active infection, which warrants treatment before restarting LDN. Clinicians must recognize that Lyme disease often represents a polymicrobial infection – tick bites can transmit co-infecting agents together and cause multiple infections, but the patient may have latent viral infections reactivated or other independent infections included in their burden of illness. (Berghoff, Walter. 2012).

MCAS, hEDS, Dysautonomia and SIBO

Sarah J. Zielsdorf, MD, MS

Abstract

This is a case of a 34-year-old female with a history of Mast Cell Activation Syndrome (MCAS), Hypermobility Spectrum, and Dysautonomia who experienced years of progressive and debilitating symptoms that affected every aspect of her life. Most notably, she experienced deep bone pain, incapacitating fatigue, loss of oral tolerance with the inability to eat most foods, intolerances to chemicals, medications, and other environmental stimuli, and poor intestinal motility leading to bacterial and fungal overgrowths and severe bloating with malabsorption. Low-dose naltrexone (LDN), in addition to other dietary and lifestyle modifications and therapeutic interventions, significantly helped the patient's quality of life via subjective improvements in pain, fatigue, and sleep, and has been taken for more than four years with sustained benefit. She has also had improvements in her labs, showing a reduction in her development of autoimmunity.

Introduction

MCAS is part of a spectrum of mast cell disorders and is considered an immune disease. The estimated prevalence of MCAS is 17%, and in this author's opinion, it is highly underdiagnosed in the general population, making it a poorly understood, rarely recognized, yet common condition. Mast cells are long-lived granulocytes (type of white blood cell) produced by the bone marrow. They contain toxic granules that, when stimulated, release over a thousand pro-inflammatory mediators. Due to many possible triggers, these mast cell chemical mediators lead to multisystemic and heterogenic inflammatory and allergic manifestations, which can affect every body system. These include constitutional symptoms, dermatologic, ophthalmologic, otologic, oropharyngeal, lymphatic, pulmonary, cardiovascular, gastrointestinal, genitourinary, musculoskeletal, neurologic, psychiatric, metabolic, hematologic, and immunologic systems

Due to poor recognition and even lack of validation in the allergy/immunology academic community, patients often suffer for up to decades with symptoms. Patients see a variety of specialists and, often due to medical trauma, stop reporting symptoms and are at risk of being diagnosed with a somatization disorder or accused of fictitious illness. MCAS itself is associated with various neurologic and psychiatric conditions, further compounding patient care. (Weinstock LB, Nelson RM, Blitshteyn S, 2023). Gastroenterologist Dr Leonard Weinstock, in addition to MCAS research with numerous published case studies, has also sought to standardize the diagnosis of MCAS via a validated Mast Cell Mediator Release Syndrome Questionnaire (MCMRS). (Weinstock LB, Brook JB, Walters AS, Goris A, Afrin LB, Molderings GJ, 2021). Research into the association of MCAS with other comorbid conditions has led to several theories, one of which is the RCCX Theory, developed by physician Dr Sharon Meglathery. (Meglathery MD, 2015). Dr Meglathery's work suggests a susceptibility in variations in the RCCX region on chromosome 6p21, which include genes such as complement component C4, CYP21 (steroid 21-hydroxylase), and TNX (tenascin-X) all of which are involved in immunity, connective tissue integrity, and endocrine pathways. Furthermore, gene alteration by chronic stress can further cause predisposition to the development of a wide range of chronic medical conditions, including but not limited to autoimmune diseases, psychiatric conditions, chronic fatigue syndrome, hypermobility, and MCAS.

Patient Description

A 34-year-old female with a past medical history significant for weight loss, loss of oral tolerance, chronic intestinal malabsorption, and chronic trauma presented to our clinic with complaints of worsening bloating, food intolerance, rashes, hives, bone pain, hair loss, and fatigue.

Case History

The patient presented to our clinic in February of 2021. Her symptoms began in September of 2019, but prior to this, due to increasing GI concerns, she became a vegetarian in 2017, followed by veganism in 2019. In the previous 3 years, she had increasing sensitivity to influenza vaccines marked by injection site reactions followed by facial flushing and heat and acute anxiety. The facial flushing persisted since then. By November 2019, she experienced shortness of breath when taking a shower or climbing a few stairs.

While peak flow readings and response to albuterol were consistent with asthma, inhaler use caused nausea, itching, and hives, for which she was successfully treated with oral steroids, but the facial rash persisted. She was then diagnosed with vocal cord dysfunction by an allergist; her steroids and inhalers were discontinued. A nasal spray, Azelastine, was prescribed to reduce post-nasal drip but caused a severe burning sunburn-like rash across the face, neck, and chest. The patient denied any use of new products or foods. Bloodwork and patch testing were negative for all food and environmental allergies, but patch testing showed contact dermatitis in response to 6-8 household chemicals. Simultaneously, additional symptoms included likely silent reflux due to hiatal hernia.

She endorsed constant bloating with significant abdominal distention and tenderness ("I looked about six months pregnant"), though she maintained her usual slight frame of 120 pounds, with chronic exhaustion and early satiety. Other symptoms included constant throat clearing, stabbing pains under the left ribcage, and constant nausea. Symptoms escalated during the COVID-19 pandemic with fevers, facial rashes, nausea, bloating, and fatigue, and new symptoms, including anxiety, tachycardia, and rashes throughout her body after taking showers and increasing body pain affecting her bones. Elimination of environmental chemicals did not help.

The patient saw a physician who suspected MCAS/SIBO (small intestinal bacterial overgrowth) and adjusted her hiatal hernia, bringing relief and the ability to breathe better and stand straighter, and no further reflux symptoms. Constipation was suspected, though the patient endorsed regular bowel movements. The patient was put on many prescription-grade supplements and a strict elimination diet after experiencing her throat closing up after eating potato salad. She avoided gluten, corn, wheat, dairy, soy, and more, sometimes fasting from all food except white rice. She was able to lose 12 pounds of bloating and felt better, had fewer reactions, but was only able to reintroduce a few foods. She continued to lose weight precipitously, eventually dropping below 110 pounds and reacting to nearly all foods except for white rice and rice cakes, quinoa, lentil pasta, carrots, broccoli, cauliflower, squashes, almond milk, olive oil, vegan butter, and salt. She was previously lactose intolerant. The patient was referred to a rheumatologist without any resultant diagnosis made.

Her immune responses did not improve, and in fact, she reacted more to other foods and continued having throat tightness and rashes, and hand eczema. Her history also included a tonsillectomy with frequent sinus infections afterward and numerous courses of antibiotics, three gum grafts due to gum recession, and an allergic reaction to Amoxicillin. Prior to establishing care, her gastroenterologist treated her gut with 1 round (2 weeks) of Rifaximin for bacterial overgrowths, which helped her bloating somewhat.

Throughout her life, she has endured many significant traumas and stressors.

In 2019 the patient experienced an ectopic pregnancy with rupture and required emergency surgery. Her body went into shock, and she nearly died. She lost one fallopian tube. In addition, she had a myomectomy for a large 10cm fibroid and difficult recovery, after which her bloating started. Since the abdominal surgeries, periods have become heavier and more painful. She grew up in suburban Chicago within a few miles of a plant accused of causing environmental contamination (ethylene oxide) and there were known cancer clusters in the community. Her mother died of aggressive breast cancer at 35, her younger brother died due to renal failure, and her father was an alcoholic who was physically abusive to her mother. The mother lost custody of the children, and so she was raised by her grandmother, who was emotionally abusive. She endorses continued toxicity in these relationships. Her father died just before establishing care. She continues to receive exposure to radiation and contrast due to increased breast cancer surveillance. Her stress levels have been constantly elevated during her training, including doctoral work and certification exams, with other requirements still pending. However she has a healthy relationship with her husband, who is supportive in every way.

Physical or Psychiatric Examination Results
Significant physical findings in 2020 included a thin woman with cracked and bleeding hands, dry skin, and significant abdominal distention. Scattered red patches and rashes across her face were present, without frank malar rash. Hypermobility was suspected due to the presence of TMJ dysfunction and open bite, and a plan for formal evaluation was made. There were no focal neurological deficits.

Test Results

Initial labs from outside clinicians in 2020 revealed a normal upper endoscopy, with a delay in SIBO testing, which revealed hydrogen-predominant SIBO on breath testing; H. pylori testing was negative. Tryptase, chromogranin-A, 24-hour urine histamine, and other metabolites were normal. Antinuclear Antibody (ANA) titer of 1:160 with normal complement proteins and normal inflammatory markers (C-Reactive Protein and Erythrocyte Sedimentation Rate). Echocardiogram was normal. Since 2020, she has had persistently low ferritin levels after one blood donation – she never recovered. A different outside clinician performed stool and food sensitivity testing, which showed Candidal (yeast) overgrowths and low levels of favorable commensal flora (poor gut bacterial diversity).

Treatment Plan

Initial management focused on reducing supplement burden, taking only essential medication and supplements to deal with sensitivities. LDN was started immediately at 0.5 mg, increasing as tolerated every 2 weeks. We focused on specific strategies to reduce immune system activation, especially at the mucosal immune system level in the GI tract with the use of serum bovine immunoglobulins to bind microbial antigens crossing a damaged gut epithelial lining that causes systemic immune activation and an inflammatory response. We dosed heavily with short-chain fatty acids, including butyrate, to support oral tolerance and improve her own probiotic microbial diversity. Optimization of magnesium and electrolyte balance was a priority. We prescribed a variety of physical therapies utilizing clinicians trained in abdominal visceral manipulation, myofascial release, and specialty care of hypermobile patients. The patient also learned abdominal self-massage techniques to work on the chronic scar tissue causing lack of blood flow (ischemia) and severe abdominal pain.

Trauma-informed and grief counseling referrals were made, and stress mitigation continues to be a focus of her treatment plan. This includes reduction of sympathetic nervous system dominance via vagal nerve stimulation exercises, including meditation, breathing exercises, and heart rate variability monitoring with biofeedback techniques.

Systemic prescription and over-the-counter antihistamine medications were added one at a time and assessed for tolerance and efficacy. The patient's current regimen includes compounded ketotifen 2 mg twice daily (2nd generation H1 receptor blocker and mast cell stabilizer), scheduled cetirizine (2nd generation H1 blocker) and famotidine (H2 blocker) twice daily, and additional mast cell stabilizer cromolyn titrating up to max dose 2 vials before meals and at bedtime. Diphenhydramine (Benedryl) is used sparingly for reactions. The patient had reactions to fexofenadine (Allegra) and nasal treatments Azelastine and Flonase. The patient found Xyzal and cyproheptadine ineffective. The patient noted the benefits of LDN, gut support including digestive enzymes and short chain fatty acids (butyrate), treatment of SIBO and SIFO (small intestinal fungal overgrowths) with repeated rounds of Rifaximin combined with herbs and proteolytic enzymes to disrupt microbial biofilms, at least one round of Nitazoxanide (an antiparasitic medication used off-label for SIBO), and prescription prokinetic medication (Prucalopride). Split dosing of LDN was utilized, working up to a higher dose given malabsorption and overgrowths. Use of estrogen metabolism support such as DIM (di-indolylmethane) to further reduce histamine burden was helpful. She was also given iron infusions with premedication for anaphylaxis prevention, which has greatly improved her quality of life.

In 2023, more than five years after the initiation of symptoms, the patient underwent consultation with Dr Lawrence Afrin, a Hematologist-Oncologist and MCAS specialist. She underwent upper endoscopy at Yale New Haven hospital. The specialty CD117+ staining of her duodenal (small intestine) and stomach biopsies were each positive for upwards of 70 mast cells/40x high-power field, and Dr Afrin confirmed the presence of mast cell activation disease in the patient.

Expected Outcome

The expected treatment outcome is improved quality of life with reduced pain and inflammation on low-dose naltrexone and control of underlying chronic mast cell symptoms.

Actual Outcome

Prior to the patient's LDN use, she described her pain as severe, unrelenting, and systemically affecting her bones, associated with crushing fatigue and slow GI motility. This is in addition to more than 40 other symptoms that originated in the fall of 2019 and increased in severity, peaking in May of 2020. She was prescribed LDN in January 2021. The intensity of her fatigue made her barely able to function in life; she described her husband struggling to wake her in the mornings, and it would take her hours to get her brain to focus each day, causing chronic lateness to work for more than a year.

Additionally, even though she experienced excruciating, deep bone pain due to her MCAS, she could not tolerate any pain medication. She reported that none of the remedies—movement, Epsom salt baths, heating pads, positioning, or any other modality—could alleviate the bone pain until she was on LDN for a few months. The pain affected her sleep, mood, concentration, and activity level. It migrated to different locations (femur, rib, collar bone, wrist, jaw) every few days, which also made life unpredictable and hard to manage. The slow motility (due to MCAS, SIBO, inflammation, surgery with subsequent adhesion and scar tissue formation, and likely more) caused severe daily bloating to the extent that the patient wore maternity underwear and pants for years.

LDN titration was well tolerated from 0.5 mg to 4.5 mg, increasing by 0.5 mg every 2 weeks. After a few months, the patient noted a decrease in her bone pain. After taking 4.5 mg for several months, she increased to 4.5 mg twice daily, which helped her general pain even more, as well as motility/bloating issues. After an extended period of time, her LDN dose was increased to 6 mg twice daily due to suspected malabsorption of medication. Her dosing of 6 mg twice daily seems to be her optimal or "maximally effective dose – MED" as coined by Dr Norman Marcus, which has further helped to resolve most of her crushing daily chronic fatigue. (Marcus NJ, Robbins L, Araki A, et al., 2024).

Furthermore, her laboratory markers have stabilized, including a reduction in ANA titers, stable immune system function, and lack of inflammation in biomarkers.

Conclusion
This case highlights the use of LDN as a fundamental therapeutic agent in the management of chronic illness for this patient with MCAS, hypermobility, dysautonomia, chronic pain, and altered GI motility/SIBO. There is a well-known common association of SIBO with either hydrogen or methane predominance or both in MCAS patients. MCAS itself can predispose patients to microbial overgrowths due to alterations in the GI immune system and altered motility due to chronic pro-inflammatory mast cell mediator release. A study of patients with refractory GI symptoms was assessed via lactulose breath test (LBT) and surveys of symptoms for the presence of MCAS and SIBO. Out of 139 MCAS subjects and 30 controls, GI symptoms preceded other MCAS symptoms in two-thirds of the cases. SIBO was present in nearly 31% of MCAS vs 10% in controls, and 83% of MCAS patients were female. In this

study, treatment of SIBO with antibiotics for 74 patients resulted in nearly 68% with marked improvement of symptoms. (Marcus NJ, Robbins L, Araki A, et al., 2024).

An additional case study of a patient with severe dysautonomia, MCAS, and SIBO responded to combination therapy, including LDN, IVIg (intravenous immunoglobulin), and antibiotics. The authors theorized that pre-existing MCAS was the driving force of the dysautonomia, characterized by severe POTS (postural orthostatic tachycardia syndrome) and hyperadrenergic autonomic nervous system activity. Antibiotic therapy with rifaximin eliminated two decades of GI symptoms. Other research has shown that a significant proportion of POTS patients have dilated and/or air-fluid levels in the small intestine, further supporting the theory that sustained sympathetic nervous system activation suppresses motility via less activation of the migrating motor complex (nerves that activate peristalsis), leading to stasis and development of SIBO. In addition, patients with concomitant hypermobility spectrum or EDS have connective tissue dysfunction leading to incompetent GI valves, including ileocecal valve integrity or droopy bowel loops. Elimination of SIBO in these patients is challenging and often requires recurrent treatment, but doing so can reduce MCAS symptoms and POTS via less intestinal permeability and reduction in immune activation, mast cell recruitment, T-cell activity, and pro-inflammatory cytokines that active mast cells. The belief that there is an autoimmune neuropathic component to this disease syndrome is supported by IVIg's mechanism of action to bind autoantibodies, and also potentially reduce mast cell mediator release or blocking histamine activation of mast cells. (Weinstock, Leonard and Brook, Jill et al., 2019).

As a reminder, histamine is a neurotransmitter that plays a role in pain perception and modulation. Furthermore, women are most frequently affected by MCAS and related syndromes. Estrogen receptors found on many immunoregulatory cells and environmental estrogens (xenoestrogens) play a role in further skewing the immune system toward allergic responses, which enhances the effects of histamine and other pro-inflammatory mediators. (Weinstock, Leonard B., Brook, Jill, et al., 2018).

MCAS requires aggressive and personalized treatment to control the symptoms caused by myriad pro-inflammatory mediator release. LDN has prokinetic activity, a mast cell stabilization effect, and is anti-inflammatory, well-tolerated, safe, and inexpensive. It should be a first-line therapeutic for all hEDS/dysautonomic/MCAS spectrum patients. In this case, the use of "High-Low Dose" Naltrexone at the dose of 6 mg twice daily had an additive beneficial effect, further reducing inflammation and overcoming the patient's intestinal malabsorption. MCAS patients benefit from LDN due to overall T-cell regulation and decreased production of cytokines, which directly cause mast cell activation. LDN also blocks Toll-like receptors (TLRs), which stimulate mast cell activity and overall reduces neuroinflammation-mediated pain via its effects on microglia. Enhanced endorphin production by LDN improves migrating motor complex activity and therefore improved GI motility, and prevention of SIBO or other microbial overgrowths. Finally, autoantibody reduction with LDN use is mediated by regulation of B-lymphocytes. (Weinstock, Leonard and Brook, Jill et al., 2018).

Mast cell disorders are highly heterogeneous and poorly understood, leading to a lack of awareness among physicians and are minimized as rare conditions. The patient's initially normal labs led to the minimization of her symptoms, medical post-traumatic stress, and reduced quality of life with the inability to gain a timely diagnosis, only to have biopsy-confirmed mast cell disease years later.

Neurological Disorders

Chronic Immune Dysregulation from Toxin Exposure

Scott Mortenson, MD

Abstract

This case study explores the use of low-dose naltrexone (LDN) in a 40-year-old male patient suffering from chronic immune dysregulation, neuroinflammation, and persistent neurological symptoms following environmental toxin exposure. The patient presented with severe cognitive impairment, chronic fatigue, gut dysbiosis, and autonomic instability, all of which worsened after prolonged mold exposure in his home. Prior treatments, including antimicrobials, antifungals, detoxification therapies, and immune modulators, provided only temporary relief. This case demonstrates how LDN was successfully incorporated into a comprehensive treatment plan, significantly improving neurological function, immune balance, and systemic inflammation.

Introduction

Chronic inflammatory and neuroimmune conditions pose significant treatment challenges, particularly when environmental triggers such as mold toxicity, chronic infections, and gut dysbiosis complicate recovery. Patients with conditions that involve persistent immune dysfunction often struggle to find effective treatments, as conventional therapies frequently fail to address the underlying drivers of neuroinflammation.

LDN has gained recognition for its ability to modulate the immune system, suppress chronic inflammation, and promote neurological recovery through its action on opioid receptors and microglial regulation. This case highlights how LDN was integrated into a broader systems-based approach to successfully reduce inflammation, stabilize immune function, and improve neurological resilience in a patient with treatment-resistant neuroimmune dysfunction.

Patient Description

The patient, a 40-year-old male computer engineer, presented with progressive neurological and systemic symptoms following long-term exposure to a mold-contaminated environment. His primary complaints included persistent brain fog, chronic fatigue, autonomic dysfunction, and gastrointestinal disturbances. He had a history of environmental sensitivities, including reactivity to chemicals, foods, and temperature changes, which had worsened over time.

History

The patient first developed symptoms in his early thirties, which were mild and episodic at first but escalated following prolonged exposure to a mold-contaminated residence. He began experiencing cognitive dysfunction, unrefreshing sleep, chemical and food sensitivities, and persistent fatigue. Despite extensive testing, he was initially misdiagnosed with anxiety and functional neurological disorder.

After several years of failed treatments, including antifungals, detox regimens, and various immune therapies, his condition remained refractory. Seeking a more comprehensive approach, he underwent advanced testing that revealed immune dysfunction, mycotoxin exposure, and persistent neuroinflammation.

Physical and Neurological Examination Results

- Cognitive Dysfunction: Severe brain fog, impaired verbal fluency, and slowed processing speed.
- Immune Dysregulation: Symptoms consistent with mast cell activation, including chemical sensitivities, histamine intolerance, and fluctuating inflammatory responses.

- Neurological Findings: Sensory hypersensitivity, autonomic instability, and mild tremors.
- Gastrointestinal Dysfunction: Chronic bloating, malabsorption, and intolerance to sulfur-containing foods, histamine and oxalates.
- Autonomic Dysregulation: Postural instability, mild tachycardia, and temperature intolerance.

Test Results
- Mycotoxin Panel: Elevated gliotoxin and trichothecenes, suggesting persistent mycotoxin burden.
- GI-MAP and OAT Tests: Confirmed gut dysbiosis, Candida overgrowth, and Clostridia-related neurotoxic metabolites.
- Neuroinflammatory Markers: Elevated oxidative stress markers, including 8-OHdG and lipid peroxides, with low glutathione levels.
- Immune Dysfunction: Positive nasal culture for MARCoNS (multiple antibiotic-resistant coagulase-negative staph), which is often linked to chronic inflammatory conditions.
- Mitochondrial Dysfunction: Low levels of key Krebs cycle intermediates, suggesting impaired energy metabolism.
- Endocrine Imbalance: Low testosterone, mild hypothyroidism, and signs of HPA-axis dysfunction.

Treatment Plan
Given the severity of immune dysfunction and neurological impairment, the treatment plan focused on stabilizing immune function, restoring mitochondrial health, and carefully integrating detoxification and neurological support.
Primary Interventions:
- T3 (5mcg BID, adjusted as needed) for metabolic and mitochondrial support.

- Enclomiphene (12.5 mg daily) to stimulate natural testosterone production.
- Plaquex IV (Phosphatidylcholine 50 mg 2x/week) for neuroprotection, cellular repair, and liver detoxification.
- MOTS-c (5 mg 3x/week) + SS-31 (5 mg daily subQ) + NAD+ IV (1-2x/week) to reverse mitochondrial dysfunction and optimize cellular energy.

Immune Modulation and Gut Repair:
- Gut Feeling (containing BPC-157, KPV, Akkermansia, and Immunolin) to repair gut permeability and regulate the immune response.
- Thymosin Alpha-1 (1.5 mg 2x/week) + LL-37 (200 mcg daily) to strengthen antimicrobial defense and reduce immune dysregulation.

Introduction of Low-Dose Naltrexone (LDN):
- Started at 0.5 mg nightly, titrated to 4.5 mg over 6 weeks.
- Goal: Reduce neuroinflammation, stabilize mast cell activity, and regulate the immune system.

Detox and Biofilm Clearance:
- BEG Nasal Spray (2x daily) + Xylitol Spray (2x daily) for MARCoNS eradication.
- Lumbrokinase (50 mg daily) + Nattokinase (100 mg daily) for biofilm disruption.
- EBOO IV (weekly, four sessions) to enhance systemic detoxification and immune function.

Neurological Repair and Cognitive Optimization:
- Semax + Cerebrolysin + Selank to restore cognitive function and neurotransmitter balance.

- Methylene Blue optional add-on.

Expected Outcome
The expected outcomes of this treatment plan included:
- Gradual reduction in neuroinflammation and cognitive dysfunction.
- Stabilization of mast cell reactivity and improved chemical and food tolerance.
- Improved mitochondrial function and energy production.
- Reduction in chronic immune activation and MARCoNS-related inflammation.

Actual Outcome
After eight weeks of treatment, the patient reported substantial improvements in:
- Cognitive clarity, with brain fog improving from a severity of 9/10 to 3/10.
- Increased energy levels, with sustained improvement in stamina and reduced post-exertional fatigue.
- Reduced histamine intolerance and chemical sensitivities.
- Improved gastrointestinal function, with less bloating and better food tolerance.

By twelve weeks, he continued to show steady improvements, with further reductions in autonomic instability and immune hypersensitivity. The integration of LDN played a critical role in stabilizing his inflammatory response, allowing other therapies to take full effect.

Conclusion
This case underscores the critical role of LDN in treating neuroimmune dysfunction and post-toxin inflammatory syndromes.

By modulating neuroinflammation, stabilizing mast cell activation, and regulating immune homeostasis, LDN contributed significantly to the patient's recovery trajectory.

Key Takeaways for Practitioners:

- LDN is most effective when introduced after foundational mitochondrial and immune support.
- Slow titration (0.5 mg to 4.5 mg over six weeks) minimizes detox flares and histamine reactions.
- LDN should be part of a systems-based approach rather than a standalone therapy.

This patient achieved measurable, sustainable improvements by incorporating LDN within a broader functional medicine framework, demonstrating its potential as a cornerstone therapy in complex neuroimmune conditions.

Trigeminal Neuritis as a Result of MCAS

Leonard Weinstock, MD, FACG

Abstract

A 54-year-old woman presented with a diagnosis of trigeminal neuralgia. She experienced severe nerve pain in the distribution of the left facial nerve for 2 years. The pain manifested as an intense burning sensation. The patient did not respond to trials of gabapentin and carbamazepine. She sought a second opinion. After taking a standard medical history and conducting a review of systems, it was revealed that she suffered from chronic diffuse body pain (fibromyalgia), restless leg syndrome, tinnitus, brain fog, fatigue, migraine, abdominal bloating, chronic non-allergic rhinitis, interstitial cystitis, and multiple food allergies. Subsequently, she was diagnosed with trigeminal neuritis caused by mast cell activation syndrome. She tapered off narcotic pain medication and switched to low-dose naltrexone (4.5 mg). There was marked improvement in her facial pain, and she later reported that the burning sensations on the top of her scalp also ceased.

Introduction

Neuropathic pain can occur anywhere in the body and often results in a poor quality of life. (Girach, Ayesha, et al., 2019). Typical cases of trigeminal neuralgia (TN) are classified as primary—either classical or idiopathic—depending on the extent of neurovascular contact. Alternatively, they may be considered secondary, arising from pathologies unrelated to neurovascular contact. (Bendtsen, L. et al., 2019) The secondary cases are often idiopathic. Classic TN manifests on one side of the face without neuropathic processes occurring elsewhere. Magnetic resonance imaging (MRI), utilizing a combination of three high-resolution sequences, is conducted as part of the assessment for TN patients. Neurovascular contact or nerve compression significantly contributes to the development of primary TN.

Medical treatment is seldom effective for this severely painful condition. The treatment approach targets general neuropathic pain relief through acute interventions with intravenous infusions of fosphenytoin or lidocaine and chronic management using carbamazepine, oxcarbazepine, lamotrigine, gabapentin, botulinum toxin type A, pregabalin, baclofen, and phenytoin. When medications fail to provide relief, neuroablative radiation treatment is the preferred option if MRI does not indicate neurovascular contact. Microsurgical interventions can alleviate vascular compression of the nerve. Treatment for patients with secondary TN involves nonspecific general neuropathic pain relief, and if this proves ineffective, the nerve may be destroyed with neuroablative radiation treatment.

The case presented herein addresses a case where a patient was diagnosed with secondary trigeminal neuralgia. Ultimately, she was diagnosed with mast cell activation syndrome (MCAS). She had multiple areas of nerve pain, and thus, the diagnosis was changed from trigeminal neuralgia to trigeminal neuritis. Mast cell-directed therapy was effective in treating facial and head nerve pain and other MCAS symptoms.

Patient Description
The patient was a well-kempt 54-year-old woman with a chief complaint of left-sided facial pain that was burning in nature and kept her awake owing to the pain. She was otherwise healthy-appearing.

History
A review of records and the taking of a careful history led to a prior diagnosis of a variety of syndromes: irritable bowel, interstitial cystitis, and fibromyalgia. Restless legs syndrome and tinnitus were

previously diagnosed and are known to be common co-morbid problems of MCAS. Other highly severe symptoms included bloating, constipation, food reactions, insomnia, migraines, rhinitis, and hives with a variety of foods. Mast cell-directed therapy was instituted.

She returned 6 months later and reported that her face pain improved entirely along with her burning scalp. She noted that cold weather was a trigger for her widespread symptoms. Her brain fog improved, and she was advised to take nasal cromolyn for additional help with her runny nose and brain fog.

On the next visit, 5 months later, her fatigue had worsened owing to an infection with COVID. She was advised to restart famotidine, which she stopped, and return to twice-daily fexofenadine, which she also did on her own. Further attempts to improve nerve symptoms in the legs with luteolin were advised. With LDN, the trigeminal neuritis remained in remission.

10-months later, she was significantly better overall, but she was trying to recover from a foot fracture that required a metal plate and screws. The implanted metal devices were tender.

Physical Examination Results
During the first examination, light palpation of the skin over the left facial nerve was incredibly tender. Palpation of the arms, legs, and shoulders muscles led to tenderness. The vital signs were normal. The joint exams were normal. The breast implants appeared normal without shift or signs of leakage.

Test Results
Two years before coming to the author's office, the MRI scan of the brain was normal. Work up by the author included mast cell mediators. The plasma histamine level was elevated at 1.9 (normal is less than 1.8). The tryptase, chromogranin A, and prostaglandin

levels were normal. The lactulose breath test revealed intestinal methane overgrowth. Ultrasound determined that the breast implants were intact.

Treatment Plan
Maintain LDN, antihistamines, linaclotide for constipation as needed, montelukast, luteolin, vitamin C, and vitamin D. Obtain metal testing to determine if the metal devices in the foot should be removed.

Expected Outcome
It is expected that she will have a good outcome. She was last seen 1 month ago. She may have a good overall outcome if the metal needs to come out of the foot.

Actual Outcome
Her facial pain showed significant improvement, and she later shared that the burning sensations on her scalp and the brain fog had both disappeared. Moreover, the patient is no longer reliant on narcotic pain medication, leading to a much-enhanced quality of life.

Conclusion
Trigeminal neuropathy is characterized by pain and numbness in the region innervated by the trigeminal nerves. Trigeminal neuropathy is most often caused by nerve compression.(Chan, Michael D., et al., 2013). Trigeminal neuritis is a form of trigeminal neuropathy in which the lesion is caused by inflammation. MCAS was the cause of the inflammation in the case presented herein. Temporomandibular joint disorders (TMJ) are associated with inflammation in trigeminal neuritis – in one series, 60 of consecutive 501 subjects with TMJ had trigeminal neuritis.(Dupont, John S. 2003). It is not commonly known that MCAS patients often have Ehlers-Danlos syndrome and that the risk of TMJ is higher in Ehlers-Danlos syndrome. This

might explain the high incidence of trigeminal neuritis in Ehlers-Danlos syndrome.

Key points covered in the case report.

- Trigeminal neuritis can be caused by mast cell activation syndrome
- Mast cell activation syndrome is a multisystemic disease, and the phenotype may vary according to the variety of mediators and triggers that each individual possesses.

Suggestions and Recommendations to Medical Professionals.
A unifying diagnosis such as MCAS is considered when a complex patient presents with multiple symptoms, syndromes, and conditions.

Chronic Pain Conditions

Polyarthralgia and Fibromyalgia

Sahar Swidan, PharmD, RPh & Matthew Bennett, MD

Abstract
This case presents a near octogenarian with long-standing recalcitrant diffuse widespread pain, polyarthralgia, and fibromyalgia. After failing traditional pharmaceutical approaches and manual therapy approaches, she obtained rapid improvement in pain and physical function with low-dose naltrexone.

Introduction
Fibromyalgia syndrome (FMS) is a disorder characterized by widespread musculoskeletal pain accompanied by fatigue, sleep disturbances, memory issues, and mood changes. In general, the primary symptom of fibromyalgia is chronic, diffuse pain. The pain must occur on both sides of your body and above and below your waist. The pain is often described as a constant dull ache lasting longer than 3 months. Frequently, overwhelming fatigue despite sufficient sleep is reported. Cognitive difficulties are commonly described as brain fog or "fibro fog." Associated conditions such as irritable bowel syndrome, migraine and other types of headaches, interstitial cystitis, anxiety, and depression are often noted.

FMS tends to run in families. According to the National Institutes of Health (NIH), several genes are thought to be associated with fibromyalgia: ADRB2 (Beta-2 adrenergic receptor), COMT (Catechol-O-methyltransferase), HTR2A (Serotonin receptor 2A), SLC6A4 (Serotonin transporter), and TAAR1 (Trace amine-associated receptor 1).

Functional MRI has shown changes in the brain with reduced grey matter volume in the pain-processing areas of fibromyalgia patients. Altered signal transmission was observed in the thalamus, indicating changed pain signaling. (Mosch, Benjamin et al., 2023). Central sensitization may play a role. Symptoms may present after a significant traumatic physical and/or psychological stress or may gradually progress over time.

This patient presented with signs and symptoms that are consistent with fibromyalgia syndrome (FMS)

Patient Description
The patient is a 79-year-old female with chronic, long-standing, diffuse widespread pain, hypertension, diabetes mellitus type two, anxiety, overactive bladder, hearing loss, and celiac disease.

History
She comes to the office with a primary complaint of significant neck pain. There is no subjective complaint consistent with cervical radiculopathy or myelopathy. Pain is fairly constant; nothing helps with the pain. She had seen some improvement with physical therapy. Upon further questioning, she admits to shoulder, back, leg, hand, and elbow pain. She has been seen by rheumatology in the past. She was diagnosed with fibromyalgia. No other clearly diagnosable autoimmune condition was found. She has tried over-the-counter anti-inflammatories, gabapentin, duloxetine, and amitriptyline without success. She cannot take acetaminophen because of allergy.

Her medications include alpha lipoic acid 100 mg daily, carisoprodol 350 mg four times a day, diazepam 5 mg every eight hours if needed for anxiety, cholecalciferol 5000 units daily, dicyclomine 10 mg four times per day, loperamide 2 mg, magnesium oxide 400 mg daily, Divalproex 250 mg daily, fluticasone proprion-salmetrol inhaled twice a day, mometasone 50 mcg inhaled daily, lisinopril 5 mg daily, clonidine 0.2 mg twice daily, metformin 500 mg twice daily, sitagliptin phosphate 100 mg daily, oxybutynin 5 mg three times a day, prednisone 10 mg twice a day.

Physical Examination Results

Physical exam showed diffuse tenderness throughout the cervical spine without a clear-cut painful structure. Normal cervical range of motion. Normal neurological exam regarding strength, sensation, and reflexes. She was wearing a thumb spica brace on the left wrist.

Imaging revealed mild disc bulging on the right greater than the left at C4-5. Mild central stenosis without cord compression at C5-6. Modic changes at C6-7. Facet spondylosis at C3-4 and C4-5 is greater than C5-6 on the left side—essentially age-appropriate changes without severe pathology.

Treatment Plan

For treatment, I talked to her about the use of low-dose naltrexone (LDN). She was intrigued by the option. I recommended that she read about low-dose naltrexone and return in 2 weeks to discuss initiation. In the meantime, she was to continue physical therapy as she found it helpful. She returned and requested the initiation of LDN. She was started at 1.5 mg daily and titrated up to 3 mg daily starting on day 10 and then 4.5 mg daily 10 days later.

Expected Outcome

The expected outcome was a gradual improvement in symptoms.

Actual Outcome

The actual outcome was a significant improvement in symptoms. Initially, she presented with 8/10 pain, primarily in the neck, but diffuse widespread pain as well. At 2 months follow-up, she had just finished the dose titration up to LDN 4.5 mg per day. The patient was tolerating the medication well without any side effects. She noted an improvement in pain to 5/10. She was feeling better enough to start a pain psychology program.

Three weeks later, she presents with pain diminished to 2/10. She continued to experience diffuse pain and polyarthralgia, but the intensity and frequency of the pain had decreased. She noted remarkable improvement in physical function and ability to ambulate despite the current time of year (spring), which is traditionally her most challenging and painful time. The next goal is to start weaning carisoprodol.

Conclusion
LDN can be a helpful and well-tolerated medication choice for patients with diffuse widespread pain, polyarthralgia, and fibromyalgia. It is typically well tolerated and without a significant side-effect profile.

Pain Management in Fibromyalgia and PMDD

Jeff Barris, PharmD & Todd Hill, ABPN

Abstract

This case study highlights an integrative approach to managing chronic pain in a patient diagnosed with fibromyalgia and premenstrual dysphoric disorder (PMDD). Presenting with severe fatigue, mental fog, joint pain, generalized pain, and weakness, the patient initially experienced adverse effects from Cymbalta prescribed for fibromyalgia. Treatment began in June 2022, focusing on Transcranial Magnetic Stimulation (TMS) and low-dose naltrexone (LDN). LDN was initiated at 0.5 mg in August 2022 and titrated to 6.5 mg, providing substantial pain relief and improved functionality. Monthly follow-ups allowed for adjustments and symptom tracking.

Additionally, Prozac was introduced to address PMDD-related symptoms, contributing to mood stabilization and reduced pain exacerbations around menstruation. The patient reported significant improvements in daily functioning and quality of life, transitioning from dependence on energy drinks to pursuing major life milestones such as marriage and planning a family. This case underscores the efficacy of multimodal pain management strategies.

Introduction

Chronic pain syndromes such as fibromyalgia are characterized by widespread pain, fatigue, cognitive dysfunction, and impaired quality of life. Fibromyalgia affects approximately 2–8% of the population, predominantly women, and remains challenging to treat due to its multifactorial nature and poorly understood pathophysiology. (Clauw, Daniel J. 2014). Conventional pharmacological treatments, including serotonin-norepinephrine reuptake inhibitors like

Cymbalta, often have limited efficacy and intolerable side effects. (Häuser, Winfried, et al., 2014). Additionally, co-occurring conditions like premenstrual dysphoric disorder (PMDD) can exacerbate pain and mood disturbances, complicating treatment plans. (Eisenlohr-Moul, et al., 2017).

Emerging therapies, such as Low-Dose Naltrexone (LDN) and Transcranial Magnetic Stimulation (TMS), have shown promise in addressing pain and enhancing neuroplasticity with fewer side effects, offering a viable alternative to conventional medications. (Younger, Jarred, et al., 2014; Lefaucheur, Jean-Pascal, et al., 2020).

The patient in this case study is a woman with fibromyalgia, who is experiencing severe pain and functional impairments, compounded by PMDD.

Patient Description
The patient is a 34-year-old female diagnosed with fibromyalgia and premenstrual dysphoric disorder (PMDD).

History
The patient initially sought treatment for severe chronic pain, fatigue, mental fog, joint and generalized pain, depression, and weakness. Her symptoms were debilitating, significantly impacting her quality of life and requiring reliance on energy drinks to function. Her pain and other symptoms worsened around her menstrual cycle, highlighting the interplay between fibromyalgia and PMDD. After experiencing adverse side effects from Cymbalta, prescribed by a rheumatologist, she sought alternative treatments.

She began receiving Transcranial Magnetic Stimulation (TMS) for depression in mid-2022 and was started on Low-Dose Naltrexone (LDN) soon after, with a titration up to 6.5 mg by 2023. Her treatment also included Prozac to address PMDD symptoms. Over the course of her care, she experienced significant improvements in pain, energy, and functionality, enabling her to achieve personal milestones, including marriage and planning for a family.

This case study explores the successful integrative management of chronic pain in a patient with fibromyalgia and premenstrual dysphoric disorder (PMDD). The focus is on addressing severe pain, fatigue, and functional impairments using a combination of low-dose naltrexone (LDN), Transcranial Magnetic Stimulation (TMS), and Prozac. The study examines the interplay between fibromyalgia and PMDD, the impact of multimodal therapies on pain and quality of life, and the patient's progression from debilitating symptoms to achieving personal and life goals. This case illustrates how nontraditional and tailored treatment approaches can effectively relieve complex chronic pain syndromes when conventional treatments fail.

Physical or Psychiatric Examination Results

Physical examination results were as follows: Pain was expressed as widespread musculoskeletal pain consistent with fibromyalgia. She experienced extreme fatigue and weakness that affected her ability to conduct daily activities properly. Psychiatric examination results were as follows: There were depression symptoms expressed through persistent low mood, mental fog, and lack of motivation as a result of experiencing pain and fatigue.

Test Results

Genetic testing consistent with a probable diagnosis of fibromyalgia. Thyroid studies, blood panels, and metabolic panels were normal. The mental status exam was consistent with major depression.

Treatment Plan

The patient's treatment plan focused on addressing chronic pain, fatigue, depression, and symptoms related to fibromyalgia and PMDD through a multimodal and integrative approach:

Low-dose naltrexone (LDN), Initiation and Titration:
* Started at 0.5 mg in August 2022, likely titrated up in increments.
* Reached 4.5 mg by October 2022 and 6.5 mg by 2023.
* Purpose: To reduce pain and inflammation and improve overall function associated with fibromyalgia.

Transcranial Magnetic Stimulation (TMS):
* Timeline: Initiated shortly after the patient's initial visit in June 2022.
* Purpose: To manage depression and potentially improve pain perception by enhancing neuronal functioning.
* The patient underwent 36 TMS treatments that were given 5 days a week and received (1) round of TMS treatments.

Prozac (Fluoxetine):
* Purpose: To manage PMDD symptoms, including mood fluctuations and increased pain severity around the menstrual cycle.Complemented other treatments by stabilizing mood and mitigating emotional triggers for pain exacerbations.

Dextroamphetamine:
* Purpose: To treat fatigue, depression, and underlying ADHD symptoms. Regular reassessing depression, energy levels, motivation, and overall mental health using patient feedback and clinical evaluations.

Follow-Up and Monitoring:
* Bi-weekly and Monthly Appointments to monitor symptom progression, adjust medication dosages, and address any side effects.

- Regular reassessing pain levels, energy, and mental health using patient feedback and clinical evaluations.

Expected Outcome

The treatment plan aimed to achieve the following outcomes for the patient.

Pain Reduction:

Significant alleviation of chronic pain, including joint and generalized pain associated with fibromyalgia, through the anti-inflammatory and neuromodulatory effects of low-dose naltrexone (LDN) and the neuroplasticity benefits of Transcranial Magnetic Stimulation (TMS).

Improved Energy and Functionality:

- Increased physical energy levels, reducing dependence on energy drinks to manage daily tasks.
- Enhanced ability to engage in routine activities and personal milestones with less fatigue and mental fog.

Mood Stabilization:

- Stabilization of mood fluctuations associated with premenstrual dysphoric disorder (PMDD), improving emotional well-being, and mitigating pain exacerbations related to hormonal changes.

Mental Clarity and Cognitive Function:

- Reducing mental fog, enhancing focus, memory, and cognitive functioning, and improving the overall quality of life.

Improved Quality of Life:

- Empowering the patient to achieve significant life goals, such as marriage and planning a family, reflecting an overall improvement in her physical and mental health.

- Ability to taper off current medications and continue with LDN for management of pain and other related symptoms.

The plan aimed for long-term symptom management, increased resilience, and a shift from daily coping to thriving in her personal and professional life.

Actual Outcome

The patient experienced significant improvements in her physical and mental health as a result of the integrative treatment plan:

Pain Reduction:

- The patient reported substantial relief from the chronic pain associated with fibromyalgia, primarily due to the effects of low-dose naltrexone (LDN). Pain exacerbations around her menstrual cycle were also mitigated, indicating improved overall symptom control.

Improved Energy and Functionality:

- Energy levels increased dramatically, enabling her to discontinue reliance on energy drinks for daily functioning. She could engage in routine activities more efficiently and maintain her energy throughout the day.

Mood Stabilization:

- Prozac effectively managed the mood fluctuations and emotional distress caused by PMDD. Combined with LDN and TMS, this contributed to improved emotional resilience and reduced pain sensitivity.

Enhanced Cognitive Function:
- The patient reported significant improvements in mental clarity and reduced cognitive fog, allowing her to navigate daily responsibilities and personal challenges better.

Improved Quality of Life:
- The patient achieved significant personal milestones, including getting married and planning to start a family later in the year. These accomplishments reflect a marked improvement in her overall quality of life and functionality.
- Due to the benefits that LDN provides, the patient is now weaning off all medications except for the LDN and is planning on starting a family.

The treatment plan successfully addressed her pain, fatigue, and depression, transforming her from a state of daily struggle to one of empowerment and hope for the future.

Conclusion

This case study illustrates the successful integrative management of a patient with fibromyalgia and premenstrual dysphoric disorder (PMDD), highlighting the importance of personalized, multimodal treatment approaches for chronic pain conditions.

Key Points from the Case Report

Challenges and Symptoms:
- The patient presented with debilitating chronic pain, fatigue, cognitive fog, and mood fluctuations, worsened by PMDD.
- Initial treatment with Cymbalta led to adverse effects, necessitating alternative therapies.

Treatment Plan:
- A multimodal approach incorporating low-dose naltrexone (LDN), Transcranial Magnetic Stimulation (TMS), and Prozac was implemented.
- Monthly follow-ups ensured symptom tracking and dosage adjustments.

Outcomes:
- Significant reduction in pain, fatigue, and PMDD-related mood fluctuations.
- Improved energy, cognitive clarity, and functionality enabled the patient to achieve personal milestones like marriage and family planning.

Suggestions and Recommendations for Medical Professionals
Adopt Integrative Treatment Approaches:
- Combine therapies like LDN and TMS to address chronic pain and psychological symptoms holistically, especially in complex conditions like fibromyalgia.

Tailor Treatment to the Individual:
- Personalize care plans based on patient-specific symptoms, coexisting conditions, and treatment responses, focusing on quality of life.

Leverage Regular Monitoring:
- Schedule consistent follow-ups to monitor progress, adjust treatments, and address emerging concerns.

Educate Patients:
• Inform patients about innovative therapies and involve them in decision-making to improve adherence and outcomes.

Consider Comorbid Conditions:
• Account for coexisting disorders like PMDD that can exacerbate symptoms and influence the effectiveness of pain management strategies.

This case underscores the value of patient-centered care and demonstrates how thoughtful, multifaceted treatment plans can significantly improve outcomes for individuals with chronic pain and associated conditions.

Autonomic Dysfunction in Long COVID

Harpal Bains, MBBS, DFSRH, PGCAestMed (Dist)

Abstract

This case highlights the challenges of managing long COVID and associated autonomic dysfunction in a 47-year-old male. Presenting with symptoms of nerve pain, skin inflammation, and circulation issues triggered by stress, the patient sought multidisciplinary care but achieved limited success. Initial interventions included lifestyle modifications and low-dose naltrexone (LDN), which provided significant pain relief and improved sleep over time. This case underscores the potential of LDN as a therapeutic option in managing chronic symptoms linked to long COVID and autonomic dysfunction.

Introduction

Long COVID presents with diverse symptoms, including nerve pain, autonomic dysfunction, and systemic inflammation. Literature suggests a possible overlap with conditions like Ehlers-Danlos syndrome (EDS) and postural orthostatic tachycardia syndrome (POTS), further complicating diagnosis and management. This case involves a 47-year-old male with chronic nerve pain and circulation issues post-COVID, demonstrating the therapeutic potential of LDN for symptom management.

Patient Description
- Age: 45 years
- Profession: Lawyer with a high-stress lifestyle
- Allergies/Sensitivities: None reported
- Family History: Mother with Parkinson's disease

History

Initial Symptoms (COVID):

- Contracted COVID-19 2.5 years ago, experiencing flu-like symptoms, cough, chest discomfort, fatigue, and loss of smell.
- Post-recovery: Circulation issues, "COVID toes," and nerve pain began, initially triggered by stress and later becoming pervasive.

Subsequent Symptoms:

- Nerve pain affecting feet and occasionally the entire body.
- Skin inflammation, especially on the face.
- No reported significant fatigue but persistent autonomic dysfunction symptoms.

The patient was diagnosed with possible Ehlers-Danlos syndrome (EDS) and autonomic dysfunction. He consulted multiple specialists, including a cardiologist, neurologist, rheumatologist, dermatologist, and allergist, but no abnormalities were found in the tests conducted.

Physical Examination Results

Key Findings:

- Pain localized to nerves, worsened with stress.
- Inflammation visible on facial skin.

Test Results

- Extensive investigations by the patients specialists yielded no abnormalities.
- Negative antibodies for autoimmune conditions.

Medications Before Coming to our Clinic:

- Amlodipine for circulation symptoms (e.g., Raynaud-like).
- Amitriptyline for nerve pain and sleep support.

- Supplements: L-theanine for relaxation and sleep.

Current Treatment Plan
Medications:
- Low-dose naltrexone (LDN): Gradual titration starting at three drops (1.5 mg) and increasing to 9 drops (4.5 mg).

Supplements:
- Magnesium and continue with L-theanine for relaxation.
- Vitamin D supplementation.

Lifestyle Modifications:
- Meditation and mindfulness exercises.
- Implementation of tapping and breathwork techniques.
- Health coaching is provided to guide the patient throughout his journey, especially in navigating any potential side effects of starting LDN. This was particularly relevant as the patient was about to give up due to side effects at certain points

Expected Outcome
- Reduction in nerve pain intensity and frequency.
- Improved sleep quality and relaxation.
- Enhanced overall well-being with reduced stress sensitivity.

Actual Outcome
Follow-Up (month 3):
- Improvement in pain with milder episodes of nerve pain.
- Severe nausea on six drops of LDN subsided after dosage adjustment to 3 drops.
- Continued vivid dreams with evening doses of LDN.

Follow-Up (month 4):
- Significant improvement in pain and reduced nausea.
- Titrated to 6 drops with slow monthly increases.

Follow-Up (month 10):
- No side effects reported
- Marked improvement in sleep and pain management, with LDN acting as a "painkiller"
- Incorporating mindfulness practices like tapping (Emotional Freedom Technique or EFT) and breathwork

Follow-Up (month 13):
- On nine drops of LDN nightly
- Better, more restful, sleep, reduced nighttime pain, and relaxation after LDN intake
- No current side effects

He continues with his current regimen, and we are considering trialling a twice-a-day LDN regime in time, which the patient is keen to try once he is further along in his journey.

Conclusion

This case illustrates the utility of low-dose naltrexone (LDN) in managing chronic pain and autonomic symptoms associated with long COVID. Gradual titration of LDN improved nerve pain, sleep quality, and overall well-being.

Stress management through mindfulness exercises complemented the pharmacological approach, highlighting the importance of a multidisciplinary strategy for such complex cases.

Clinicians should consider LDN for patients with similar chronic symptoms, especially when conventional treatments yield limited results.

Chronic Cervical Radiculopathy in a 32-Year-Old
Greta Niemela, MD & Neel Mehta, MD

Abstract
We present a case of a 32-year-old male suffering from neck and arm pain, muscle spasms, and numbness who failed conservative management and was not a surgical candidate. He had a working diagnosis of chronic cervical radiculopathy. He has had a positive response to 6 mg of low-dose naltrexone (LDN), and his symptoms have been well controlled for more than one year.

Introduction
Chronic pain is one of the most significant public health problems in the United States. Often, patients have tried many treatment modalities without significantly relieving their symptoms. Though naltrexone has been available for decades in the United States, it has traditionally been used as a treatment for substance use disorders. More recently, LDN has emerged as a novel and safe option to treat a variety of chronic pain conditions. However, research has focused on fibromyalgia. Here, we present a case of a patient with a history of C3-4 disc herniation complicated by chronic neck pain, spasms, and numbness that is refractory to traditional pharmacological interventions and epidural steroid injections.

Patient Description
The patient is a 32-year-old male with a history of intermittent gastroesophageal reflux (GERD) addressed through diet control and occasional low back pain and muscle spasms that resolved without intervention over the past 15 years. He presented to our outpatient pain clinic with severe chronic neck pain for 3 years that began suddenly while he was changing his clothing. The pain was associated with spasms, numbness, and weakness at the base of his

neck on the right side, which were worse with certain positions. Additionally, he reported weakness in his right 2nd and 3rd fingers that had since resolved.

History
One year after the onset of the pain, the patient participated in 9 months of physical therapy followed by a home exercise program that was ongoing at the time of presentation. Several medications were tried, including pregabalin, which provided no benefit, and non-steroidal anti-inflammatory drugs (NSAIDs) and cyclobenzaprine muscle relaxant, which provided only minor relief. These medications were stopped due to the lack of benefits and contraindications of NSAIDs and GERD. Additionally, he received two cervical C3/C4 epidural steroid injections, each of which provided significant relief of the numbness of the fingers but only mild improvement in the pain for approximately 6 weeks.

Physical Examination Results
The physical exam was notable for moderate tenderness to palpation around cervical paraspinal muscles, notable paraspinal muscle spasm, and his right shoulder was elevated. Neurologically, his strength was intact in his upper extremities. He had a negative Spurling test. He was negative for hypermobility on the Beighton Scale (0 of 9).

Test Results
The patient had undergone several imaging studies about 1.5 years prior to presentation. An X-ray of the cervical spine showed a slight coronal curve, C2-C7 kyphosis of 12 degrees, and local kyphosis at C5-6 with mostly preserved disc height. MR cervical spine was significant for large paracentral right disc herniation impinging cord and causing mild central stenosis at C3-C4, mild left foraminal

stenosis at C4-5, and central disc protrusion contacting cord, mild central stenosis, and mild left foraminal stenosis at C5-6. CT cervical spine was significant for posterior osteophytes at C5-6, kyphosis at C3-4 and C5-6. The patient also underwent an EMG that was negative for active cervical radiculopathy on the right.

Treatment Plan
The patient was evaluated for cervical spine surgery and was found not to be a candidate unless he failed conservative management. Given the prior treatments of NSAIDs, pregabalin, and cyclobenzaprine, the patient started on low-dose naltrexone at 0.1 mg and was slowly titrated up over 3 months to a final dose of 6 mg daily. Also, the patient was prescribed a topical compounded lidocaine and ketamine cream to use as needed, but he found less benefit. He also continued his physical therapy program.

Expected Outcome
The patient was seeking non-surgical options and had failed conventional and conservative treatments. He had not previously heard of LDN. It was expected that the LDN, paired with continued physical therapy, would improve the patient's pain symptoms and function.

Actual Outcome
Although the patient did not find benefits from lower doses of LDN, he experienced significant relief from pain symptoms at 6 mg daily. He experienced increased energy and mild nausea with the dose but could tolerate minimal side effects. He has remained on the current treatment regimen for 1 year and is highly satisfied with the improvement.

Conclusion

This case demonstrates a patient with C3-4 disc herniation with radicular neck pain and numbness that was refractory to physical therapy, epidural steroid injections, and other traditional pharmacological treatment, including pregabalin, NSAIDS, and muscle relaxants. The patient started on an LDN treatment program combined with continued physical therapy and experienced significant improvement in his symptoms with minimal side effects. This illustrates the potential therapeutic opportunity that LDN may provide in patients with chronic pain refractory to traditional management, but the dose required is particular to the patient.

Idiopathic Small Fiber Neuropathy and CRPS

Meredith Kushner, MD, MS & Neel Mehta, MD

Abstract

We present a case of a 57-year-old female with a history of gastroparesis and diffuse, generalized neuropathic pain in the setting of idiopathic small fiber neuropathy with complex regional pain syndrome (CRPS) who found significant relief in pain symptoms with low-dose naltrexone (LDN). The patient experienced adverse gastrointestinal (GI) side effects on LDN 3.5 mg in the standard formulation; these side effects resolved after reducing the dose to LDN 2 mg and switching the formulation to a ginger filler.

Introduction

Naltrexone is an opioid antagonist approved to treat opioid use disorder and alcohol use disorder at a dose of 25-50 mg daily. Low-dose naltrexone (LDN) is a novel off-label dose of naltrexone used to treat chronic pain syndromes. The side effects of LDN are rare; fatigue, anxiety, and dizziness have been reported. In this case, we report on treating pain with LDN in a patient with idiopathic small fiber neuropathy with complex regional pain syndrome (CRPS), as well as managing GI side effects of LDN in the setting of underlying gastroparesis and a history of GI upset related to medications.

Patient Description

The patient is a 57-year-old female with a past medical history of asthma, chronic kidney disease, X-linked Alport syndrome in heterozygous female, gastroparesis, gallstones, thyroid nodules, endometriosis, herpes simplex, and sucrose-isomaltose disaccharidase deficiency who presents to chronic pain clinic with 2 years of diffuse, generalized neuropathic pain, most severe in bilateral lower extremities, in the setting of idiopathic small fiber neuropathy and complex regional pain syndrome (CRPS).

History

The patient's symptoms began with acute bilateral foot pain, described as burning and stabbing, that migrated superiorly with squeezing pain to the entire legs. She also experienced throbbing, burning pain in bilateral upper extremities, neck spasms, and stabbing, non-radiating pain in the lumbar spine region. She describes the pain as migratory and intermittent. Her pain was worse at night and disrupted her sleep. She reported sporadic feelings of heaviness and subjective weakness in her extremities.

Upon initial presentation, she was taking no medications for pain relief. In the past, she had tried acetaminophen, which provided limited relief, as well as gabapentin, nortriptyline, and ibuprofen, which she stopped due to adverse side effects. She describes the challenges of GI side effects due to gastroparesis.

She also follows with rheumatology, neurology, rehab medicine, and integrative medicine clinicians. She participates in physical and occupational therapy, Pilates, and massage therapy. She tried acupuncture in the past but stopped due to exacerbation of symptoms. She experienced some relief with steroid and alcohol injections into her foot with outside providers.

Physical Examination Results

The physical exam upon the initiation of LDN was notable for hypersensitivity and redness in the lower extremities. After a stable dose of LDN, the examination was normal, with minimal redness and hyperalgesia.

Test Results

Labs for contributing causes have been unremarkable.

She was evaluated by a neurologist; skin biopsies were consistent with small fiber neuropathy. She was evaluated by a rheumatologist; the workup was negative for myositis. She underwent genetic testing, which was negative. Electromyography and nerve conduction studies were unremarkable.

MRI of the brain, cervical spine, and thoracic spine showed no spinal cord abnormalities. MRI of the lumbar spine showed mild degenerative and discogenic changes at the L4-5 level, contributing to mild bilateral neural foraminal narrowing and mild bilateral facet arthropathy at L5-S1. XR pelvis showed no significant degenerative changes of the bilateral hips. XR bilateral hands showed no evidence of erosive or inflammatory arthropathy of the bilateral hands.

Treatment Plan
She was prescribed an LDN titration, starting at 0.1 mg PO daily, then adding 0.1 mg by mouth daily every 3 days until reaching a dose of 1 mg daily, with plans to titrate the LDN dose further pending tolerance and clinical response. She was also prescribed duloxetine 20 mg by mouth daily, which was then discontinued within 1 week due to adverse effects of GERD, also a topical compounded lidocaine-ketamine cream. A sympathetic block was considered; however, given her broad systemic issues, this intervention was deferred to be reconsidered in the future, pending response to medical management.

Expected Outcome
The patient had failed other conservative medication, rehabilitative, and alternative treatments. She was seeking non-surgical intervention to improve her pain and was unfamiliar with LDN before her presentation to our clinic. She expressed understanding that her small fiber neuropathy contributed to much of her pain and

was open-minded to trying LDN while continuing the management of neuropathy with her neurologist.

Actual Outcome.
The patient experienced significant relief with LDN therapy (80% symptom improvement). After 6 months of LDN 1 mg daily, the LDN dose was titrated by 0.5 mg every 2 weeks to a daily dose of 3.5 mg, where the patient experienced GI side effects due to gastroparesis and GERD while taking LDN. A liquid formulation was tried without improvement in symptoms. Her dose was decreased to LDN 2 mg, and a ginger filler formulation was tried with a resolution to adverse GI side effects.

After initiating intravenous immunoglobulin (IVIG) with her neurologist while continuing daily LDN, the patient began experiencing brief episodes of lightheadedness that she believes are temporally linked to IVIG. We recommended continuing LDN at the current dose and formulation with close follow-up and to consider dividing the 2 mg daily dose into 1 mg twice daily dose if lightheadedness symptoms persisted.

Conclusion
This case demonstrates the effectiveness of LDN in treating CRPS in small fiber neuropathy with slow titration. Additionally, this case demonstrates the effectiveness of altering the LDN formulation to ginger filler for patients experiencing GI side effects with underlying gastrointestinal disease.

Erythromelalgia: Persistent Lower Extremity Pain

Neel Mehta, MD & Arash Jalali-Sohi, Medical Student

Abstract

We present herein the case of a 45-year-old male with no significant medical history besides Raynaud's disease who presented with bilateral foot pain and erythromelalgia. The patient endorsed radicular symptoms to the feet, including numbness, tingling, and mild weakness. Continuous physical therapy for one year failed to resolve symptoms. He had previously taken gabapentin and pregabalin, which posed no benefit. NSAIDs and topical lidocaine provided minor and moderate benefits, respectively. The patient was prescribed ketamine cream and low-dose naltrexone (LDN), which was titrated from 0.1 mg to 6 mg over three months. He has tolerated side effects well and had improved mood, increased energy and reduced pain. The patient was continued on ketamine 15%/lidocaine 15% cream, LDN 6 mg/day, and physical therapy.

Introduction

Naltrexone is an opioid antagonist approved to treat opioid use disorder and alcohol use disorder at a dose of 25-50 mg daily. Low-dose naltrexone (LDN) is a novel off-label dose of naltrexone used to treat chronic pain syndromes. The side effects of LDN are rare; fatigue, anxiety, and dizziness have been reported. In this case, we report on treating pain with LDN in a patient with erythromelalgia, as well as managing GI side effects of LDN in the setting of underlying gastroparesis and a history of GI upset related to medications.

Erythromelalgia is a rare medical condition characterized by episodes of intense burning pain, redness, warmth, and swelling, typically affecting the hands and feet. The symptoms can range from mild to severe and are often triggered or worsened by heat, exercise, or other activities that increase blood flow to the affected areas.

Patient Description
The patient was seeking non-surgical options and had failed conventional and conservative treatments. He had seen several physicians with unsuccessful treatments to that point. He had not previously heard of LDN but was optimistic.

History
This 45-year-old male patient presented with bilateral foot pain and erythromelalgia, which he had suffered from for multiple years. He had no significant past medical history, except for Raynaud's disease. Continuous physical therapy for the past year did not result in any symptom improvement. The patient had previously taken gabapentin and pregabalin, but these failed to alleviate any pain. He had minor pain reduction from NSAIDs, and moderate benefits from topical lidocaine cream.

Physical Examination Results
Physical examination was notable for bilateral foot pain with itching, swelling, redness, and temperature change, as well as radicular symptoms of numbness, tingling, and mild weakness. No edema, masses, or open wounds were noted. Lower extremity strength was 5/5 and dorsalis pedis pulse was palpable bilaterally. Review of systems was otherwise unremarkable.

Test Results
An MRI of the bilateral feet and lumbar spine was unremarkable. Electromyography (EMG) and nerve conduction testing (NCT) were negative.

Treatment Plan

The patient was prescribed ketamine cream and a gradually increasing titration of LDN. The LDN was started at 0.1 mg/day and titrated up to a final dosage of 6 mg/day over three months. He was advised to continue with physical therapy as tolerated.

Expected Outcome

It was expected that LDN would reduce the inflammation evident in his feet and thereby reduce pain.

Actual Outcome

He has tolerated side effects well and had improved mood, reduced swelling and pain, and increased energy. The patient has continued on ketamine 15%/lidocaine 15% cream as needed, LDN 6 mg/day, and physical therapy.

Conclusion

We present the case of LDN treating refractory lower extremity pain and redness related to erythromelalgia. Treatment with LDN was well tolerated with minimal side effects and should be considered for this condition.

Full-Thickness Rotator Cuff Tear

Rehana Sajjad, MD, FACOG, ABAARM

Abstract
A female patient presented with a full-thickness tear of the right shoulder rotator cuff and was in considerable pain. Painkillers were providing minimal relief, and she was scheduled for surgery to attempt to reattach the tendon to the bone. In the meantime, the patient needed assistance and was placed on low dose naltrexone and other treatments to support her overall health and reduce the inflammation evident in her lab work. After two to three weeks the patient felt she could postpone her surgery due to the pain relief she experienced from the treatments I provided.

Introduction
The rotator cuff consists of four muscles and their tendons, which stabilize the shoulder joint. A full-thickness tear refers to a complete detachment of the tendon from the bone, particularly at its attachment on the humerus (upper arm bone). Symptoms include: sudden or gradual pain, weakness in the shoulder and arm, difficulty lifting or lowering the arm, a grinding or cracking sound during shoulder movement, and increased pain at night or when lying on the affected side.

Full-thickness tears can result from degenerative changes (wear and tear) over time, trauma such as a fall or impact, or repetitive movements and heavy lifting. Treatment options may involve rest, ice therapy, physical therapy, and anti-inflammatory medications. If relief is not achieved, surgical intervention may be necessary, during which the torn tendon is reattached to the bone.

Recovery duration varies based on the tear size and treatment type. A small tear might take about 4 months to recover, while larger tears can require up to 12 months.

Patient Description
The patient is a 71-year-old female. The patient presented with a full-thickness tear of the right shoulder rotator cuff and had been suffering from significant pain for 2-3 months. She experienced severe pain, often screaming in distress, and was unable to sleep more than an hour at night, with pain intensifying during the evening. Despite taking Tylenol and Advil frequently, her pain relief was minimal.

History
Her medical history includes a right mastectomy due to cancer, followed by chemotherapy and radiation. Subsequently, she developed right parotid gland cancer, which required additional surgery, radiation, and chemotherapy. These treatments have left her with notably weakened jaw bones.

Test Results
Knowing her previous case, I requested her radiology and lab reports. Her inflammatory markers were significantly elevated

Treatment Plan
Due to her inflammation, I initiated a treatment plan that included low-dose naltrexone (LDN), starting at 1.5 mg daily and gradually increasing to 4.5 mg. Additionally, I prescribed an ultimate pain block oral spray, local application, BPC-157, and magnesium malate orally, along with DMSO locally. To support her overall health, I recommended a regimen of B complex vitamins, vitamin D, vitamin K2, vitamin C, NAC, CoQ10, and liposomal curcumin.

Expected Outcome

I expected a reduction in her inflammatory markers and a reduction in her pain and therefore a far better quality of life.

Actual Outcome

After 2-3 weeks, she reported a noticeable improvement in her pain levels and ultimately became pain-free. Her orthopedic surgeon had warned that her shoulder pain might worsen and she was scheduled for surgery. However, due to a dental issue, she decided to postpone the surgery, opting to address her dental concerns first, especially since she was now pain-free. Furthermore, she noted an improvement in her other arthritic joint pains as well.

Conclusion

Pain relief can be achieved with a combination of LDN, peptides and natural supplements. This patient didn't need to suffer for the time between her injury and surgery, which could have been a prolonged wait. Lowering inflammation reduces pain by reducing pressure on the nerve endings. LDN and other anti-inflammatory supplements help to ease the

Fibromyalgia, RA, and Systemic Lupus Erythematosus

Sahar Swidan, PharmD, RPh & Matthew Bennett, MD

Abstract

This case presents a middle-aged woman with fibromyalgia and autoimmune disease who presents with a mixed pattern of diffuse pain and nociceptive spinal arthritic pain. Low-dose naltrexone can provide efficacious and durable pain relief. Side effects are minimal and can usually be addressed.

Introduction

Lymphocytes (T and B cells) play a central role in adaptive immunity by recognizing specific antigens. Lymphocytes can become reactive to native tissue. Usually, the immune system eliminates or controls self-reactive lymphocytes.However, in autoimmunity, there is defective elimination and/or control of these self-reactive lymphocytes. (Rosenblum, Michael D. et al., 2015). Genetic and environmental triggers may contribute to inciting or exacerbating autoimmune conditions.

LDN may provide potential benefits in treating autoimmune conditions. White blood cells have opioid receptors. LDN could regulate the immune system by promoting the function of T regulatory cells (Tregs) to maintain immune balance. It may decrease inflammatory cytokines (TNF-α, IL-6, IL-12 alpha, and IL-17) and increase the anti-inflammatory cytokines (IL-10). (Carvalho, Jozélio Freire de, and Thelma Skare. 2023).

In the central nervous system, chronic activation of the toll-like receptor 4 (TLR4) on the microglia results in neuroexcitotoxicity, which creates some symptoms consistent with fibromyalgia syndrome. LDN blocks TLR4.

This patient presents with pain associated with presumed autoimmunity, fibromyalgia, and nociceptive lumbar facet arthritis.

Patient Description

The patient is a 49-year-old female with long-standing lower back pain associated with facet arthritis. She has previously responded to radiofrequency ablation at L4-5 and L5-S1. She comes in complaining of return of back pain and requesting a repeat radiofrequency ablation. Upon further questioning, she admits to other painful regions. She describes a thoracic achy sensation without a clear-cut region of maximal tenderness. She has bilateral buttock and hip pain and diffuse non-dermatomal pain into the legs bilaterally. She also describes achiness in the bilateral hands. She had been tolerating this more diffuse pain reasonably well until recently without any new inciting event.

History

Thirty years ago, she was diagnosed with fibromyalgia syndrome, rheumatoid arthritis, and systemic lupus erythematosus (SLE) after developing a malar rash and pulmonary difficulties. There was also concern about possible multiple sclerosis (MS) when she developed otherwise unexplainable facial paresthesia. She has been seen by neurology and rheumatology. She has seen ophthalmology and has been treated for uveitis. She was treated with NSAIDs and opioids without significant improvement. Oral steroids were helpful but resulted in substantial weight gain. She had tried duloxetine and gabapentin without improvement.

Physical Examination Results

Her physical exam showed significant tenderness to palpation over the L4-5 and L5-S1 facet joints bilaterally. The pain worsens with extension to 10 degrees and much worse with extension and lateral rotation (Kemp test). The pain was better with forward flexion. The pain was not recreated with the hip joint range of motion, not the FABER test. Negative straight leg raising both seated and supine. The neurological exam was normal.

Imaging of her lumbar spine from 2015 showed severe facet arthritis at L4-5 and L5-S1. No significant disc pathology. No neural compression. Labs showed a negative anti-nuclear antibody (ANA), rheumatoid factor (RF), cyclic citrullinated peptide (CCP), human leukocyte antigens B27 (HLA-B27), and normal erythrocyte sedimentation rate (ESR) and C-reactive protein (CRP).

Treatment Plan

The treatment plan was discussed. We agreed to repeat the bilateral L4-5 and L5-S1 radiofrequency ablation as she previously had greater than 80% pain relief for more than six months. She knows her symptoms have flared up since changing her eating habits. She had been eating fast food and takeout because her hand pain was such that she could no longer cook and prepare food. She proposed that she get back to eating a "clean" diet by avoiding excess refined carbohydrates (including sodas) and being certain to include more vegetables. In the past, her symptoms were better with this.

I talked to her about utilizing low-dose naltrexone (LDN) for her current symptoms. After discussing risks, possible benefits, and alternatives, she wanted to proceed with low-dose naltrexone compounded, adding 1 mg per day for the first week. After this, she will titrate with one additional milligram weekly for four weeks. In the fifth week, she would increase her dose to 4.5 mg daily and stay at this dose.

Expected Outcome

The expected treatment plan was a significant improvement in lumbar spine arthritis pain and partial improvement in her diffuse symptoms.

Actual Outcome

The Actual Outcome was as follows: Six weeks later, the patient came in, stating that the LDN had "changed my life." She reported a significant improvement in her diffuse and polyarthralgia pain, and the back pain from the facet arthritis had also resolved (status post radiofrequency ablation). She was taking LDN at night and noticed sleep disturbance with disturbingly vivid dreams. We transitioned the LDN to daytime dosing, and the sleep symptoms subsided. This response to LDN was consistent with its known effects on pain relief and immune system modulation.

Two months later, the patient experienced a severe ear infection that required three weeks of oral antibiotics. This resulted in a severe flareup of her pain, as well as a severe "lupus flare" with the return of her malar rash and a severe re-exacerbation of her diffuse pain symptoms. She requested that we stop the LDN at that point as she felt discouraged by the worsening of pain. She worked on rebuilding the microbiome by taking probiotics, drinking kombucha, and eating fermented vegetables.

Six weeks after this, she noted cognitive and speech difficulties, which were worked up by neurology, and no clear diagnosis was found, although MS was considered possible. Four weeks after this, she returned to the clinic, having restarted LDN independently, and was feeling much better again. This decision to restart LDN reflects the patient's understanding of her condition and her proactive approach to managing her symptoms.

It has been 7 years since she started on LDN, and she has overall done very well with her diffuse pain and polyarthralgia. She has continued to experience tremendous benefits with radiofrequency ablation for the severe point tender lower lumbar facet arthritis pain. She is back to work in a self-owned greenhouse and organic goat's milk business, which she tends to herself. She has had intermittent flare-ups of autoimmune-type skin lesions, finger joint arthritic effusions, and uveitis. Multiple rheumatologists have not been able to diagnose an autoimmune disease definitively.

Conclusion

LDN can be a helpful choice for patients with pain consistent with fibromyalgia or autoimmune disorders. We typically co-treat with and have open discussions with rheumatology and neurology (when MS is considered). When patients experience sleep-related side effects, altering dose timing can be beneficial. LDN can lose efficacy; in this case, a short break in therapy allowed the return of durable efficacy.

Exploring an Adjunctive Therapy for Fibromyalgia

Scott Mortenson, MD

Abstract

This case study examines a 42-year-old female with fibromyalgia, characterized by chronic widespread pain and fatigue. Traditional treatments (analgesics, antidepressants) provided minimal relief. Low-dose naltrexone (LDN) was introduced to modulate inflammation and pain perception. After 12 weeks, LDN titrated from 1.5 mg to 3 mg to 4.5 mg nightly, the patient reported a 64% pain reduction and improved sleep. This suggests LDN's potential as an adjunctive therapy for fibromyalgia.

Introduction

Fibromyalgia affects 2–4% of the population, with chronic pain and fatigue as hallmark symptoms. Current treatments like NSAIDs and gabapentinoids often fall short. LDN, an opioid antagonist at low doses, has shown promise in reducing pain via immune modulation (Stanford Medicine, 2023). This case involves a 42-year-old woman with fibromyalgia and severe musculoskeletal pain.

Patient Description

A 42-year-old Caucasian female, married, with no children, works part-time as a fitness instructor.

History

Diagnosed with fibromyalgia 5 years ago after experiencing diffuse pain, fatigue, and sleep disturbances. Previous treatments included ibuprofen (minimal effect) and duloxetine (partial relief). Pain rated 7/10 on average.

Examination Results

Tender points positive at 14/18 sites—no joint swelling. Mood stable, mild anxiety noted.

Test Results

Normal blood work (CBC, CRP, ESR). Negative rheumatoid factor and ANA, ruling out autoimmune mimics.

Treatment Plan

LDN started at 1.5 mg nightly and was titrated to 4.5 mg over 4 weeks. Duloxetine continued at 60 mg daily.

Expected Outcome of the Treatment Plan

Reduction in pain by 30–50% and improved sleep within 12 weeks, based on LDN's anti-inflammatory effects.

Actual Outcome

After 12 weeks, pain decreased to 2.5/10, sleep quality improved (self-reported 8-hour sleep vs. 5-hour baseline). Mild headaches initially, resolved by week 6.

Conclusion

This case highlights LDN's potential in reducing fibromyalgia pain and improving quality of life. Medical professionals might consider LDN for refractory cases, with careful dose titration to minimize side effects.

Complex Regional Pain Syndrome

Yusuf M. Saleeby, MD, CTP

Abstract

This case report is on the use of low dose naltrexone (LDN) in assisting a patient with years of chronic pain (chronic complex regional pain syndrome [CRPS]). This case illustrates the most effective dose and, by happenstance, how this was discovered as a misunderstanding of instructions. To everyone's amazement, her pain dropped to zero (0/10 on the pain scale). LDN can be used as a solo therapy, administered twice daily (BID) 12 hours apart for better efficacy in managing pain. It can also be used in combination with cannabinoids (utilizing the ECS- endocannabinoid system) for better pain modulation/mitigation.

Introduction

This patient was a referral from a general medicine allopathic office. She was diagnosed with chronic Lyme disease (CLD) prior to our first encounter and was intolerant of allopathic therapies. She was suffering from Herxheimer reactions and came to us for better CLD management and pain control. Her primary condition was chronic or late-phase Lyme disease (Borreliosis) with chronic regional pain syndrome.

Patient Description

Patient E.C. is a 37-year-old female who presented for the first time in March 2022. Her Chief Complaint was chronic fibromyalgia and regional pain syndrome. She was also diagnosed by positive serology with Lyme disease and with rheumatoid arthritis (RA) by a rheumatologist.

History

She was seen by several medical professionals since September of 2020, when the first symptoms arose of right wrist pain. She was examined by specialists and had an injection of steroids and lidocaine in her wrist. After an IV for a CT study, the pain then "marched up her arm." Following more diagnostics and interventions, such as an injection in her neck, she then experienced bilateral arms and leg discomfort. An MRI of the head/neck was ordered, and other issues arose. MRI ruled out multiple sclerosis (MS). Specialists in neurology and rheumatology did not help make diagnoses or interventions. RA and tendonitis were diagnosed, but treatments were ineffective. Methotrexate for 6-months and Etanercept (Enbrel) injections were not effective. Hence, after suffering for over six months, she presented to us in this condition.

Past Medical history: foot surgery, Morton's neuroma, NKDA, no environmental or food allergies. Medications on presentation: she was taking Gabapentin 800 mg TID, Buprenorphine (Belduca) 900 mcg SL, Ibuprofen 800 mg PRN, Pepcid, and Zofran PRN. She has a social history of vaping and weekly wine drinking. Social history: she was in sales but is classified as disabled. Family History: BrCA, DM, skin cancer, ovarian cancer, Lupus, RA, and dementia; She was vaginally delivered and breastfed for only one week. The patient was born in New Jersey and traveled to DE, SC, West VA. She was UTD on childhood vaccines but no flu or mRNA COVID vaccine history.

At the age of 20 or so, she claims to have had a bullseye (EM) rash on her left arm. No treatment was rendered back then to cover tick-borne illness—review of systems: tinnitus, vertigo, POTS, pain 24/7, and a feeling of burning inside.

Physical or Psychiatric Examination

Alert/Oriented x4 but in obvious pain constantly. No acute distress, well developed, several tattoos, presented with mother and fiancé in the room: HEENT: WNL, no apparent abnormalities. Neck unremarkable. CV/Lungs unremarkable; CTA, RRR with no m/r/g; Abdomen: overtly normal; Ext/Skin: WNL; Neuro/Psych: A/O x 4, No depression or focal neurological findings. Adult depression screening performed: No indicators for depressive disorder. The screening was negative for fall risk or unsafe living environment.

The Rhomberg test was negative; the single-leg standing balance was not good, and the gait was normal. Motor function was 4+/5 bilateral hand strength. Labs: IGENEX + for Bb, no positive co-infections; MRI reports, etc., and other older labs reviewed.

Test Results
MRI reports negative for pathology. IGENEX-labs were positive for Bb but negative for co-infections.

Treatment Plan
On day one, we referred her out for acupuncture for pain management; we advised the cessation of alcoholic beverages. We gave information and education about the use of CBD and Delta8/ THC to reduce dependence on opiates (Buprenorphine/Belbuca); once off Belbuca, we could start LDN. Started LDN 0.5 mg caps BID (every 12 hours) once off central-acting pain meds. And titration up thereafter. Ivermectin (IVM) at 40 mg once daily with food for a trial (anti-Lyme). Use of botanicals "Banderol and Samento (Cat's claw) from NutraMedix" were also initiated and titrated up from 1-30 drops BID; Herxing information and protocols for mitigation were given. Follow-up was for 2 to 3 months.

Expected Outcome
Once weaned off the opiates, she started LDN at 1.0 mg BID and tolerated this without major ASE. She suffered some signs of opiate withdrawals on April 11th, 2022, and Herxing (J-H Herxheimer

reaction) on April 21st, 2022, as reported to nursing staff. Pain, insomnia, and diarrhea were complaints, and the Acute Pain Relief (EuroMedica) formula was added (curcumin, Boswellia serrata, ginger combo). April 28, 2022, she decided to stop Gabapentin on her own. On October 3rd, 2022, she still reported pain on a lower dose of LDN. She was now off Gabapentin. On December 1st, 2022, she was placed on Cefuroxime Axetil (Ceftin) 250 mg BID; IVM EOD; Methylene Blue very low dose of 1-drop/day 1% solution; Folate and vitamin B12; LDN at this point was increased to 4 mg BID (after a slow titration upwards);

During a visit on May 2nd, 2022 she was instructed to take 1.5 mg of LDN BID (3 mg total daily dose) however, she misunderstood the instructions and took 3 mg BID. This dose caused immediate resolution of her pain state with 0/10 pain on standard reporting pain assessment. She continued this dose of 3 mg BID from May until December of 2022 until such time as an increase was made to LDN 4 mg BID (8 mg total dose/day). This increase was because pain returned on the 6 mg/d dose. Raising to 8 mg/d was more effective.

For whatever reason, she stopped LDN on May 8th, 2023. She was lost to follow up after a visit on May 8th, 2023, for recurrence of symptoms, pain following an ocean cruise, steroid injection, and ibuprofen use for a "flare up" of her condition. We are not entirely clear as to why she stopped her LDN and most of her protocol; we will never know clearly as she stopped returning to us for care following the May 2023 visit.

Actual Outcome
Realization after many years of suffering from chronic pain and fibromyalgia that the combination of a higher than usual BID dose schedule of LDN resulted in the resolution of pain when other agents and procedures did not.

This illustrates that limiting the dose of LDN to the usual 4.5 mg/day may not work for everyone, and in some instances, higher than usual doses (up to 8 mg/day) may be more effective for pain management. Adding other agents as pain modulators/modifiers can be helpful. Add-on or adjunctive medications and/or cannabinoid therapies should be tried with each chronic pain patient.

Conclusion

A combination of a higher than usual BID (twice daily) dose schedule of low dose naltrexone (LDN) can cause resolution of pain when other agents and procedures do not. This case illustrates that limiting the dose of LDN may not work for everyone, and in certain cases, higher than usual doses (up to 8 mg/day of naltrexone) may be effective. Adding other agents, such as pain modulators/modifiers, may be helpful. Medications (such as tricyclics and botanicals) and/ or cannabinoids (CBD and other cannabinoids and terpenes) should be tried with each chronic pain patient.

LDN for Complex Regional Pain Syndrome

Pradeep Chopra, MD, MHCM

Abstract

Complex regional pain syndrome (CRPS) is a debilitating chronic pain condition characterized by severe pain, autonomic dysregulation, and sensory abnormalities. Traditional treatments often yield suboptimal results, prompting exploration of alternative therapies. This report presents the case of a 24-year-old female diagnosed with CRPS who experienced significant symptomatic improvement following treatment with low-dose naltrexone (LDN).

Introduction

CRPS is a neuropathic pain disorder that typically follows trauma, surgery, or other inciting events. Current treatment options include physical therapy, pharmacotherapy, and interventional procedures, but many patients continue to experience significant morbidity. Emerging evidence suggests that LDN, an opioid antagonist with anti-inflammatory and immunomodulatory properties, may offer a novel therapeutic approach.

Case Presentation

A 24-year-old previously healthy female presented with severe burning pain, hyperalgesia, and allodynia in her right lower extremity following a minor ankle sprain. Over several weeks, her symptoms progressed to include swelling, temperature dysregulation, and significant functional impairment. Clinical examination and diagnostic testing confirmed a diagnosis of CRPS Type I based on the Budapest Criteria. According to these criteria, CRPS is diagnosed when a patient exhibits continuing pain disproportionate to any inciting event and at least one symptom in three of the four following categories: sensory (hyperalgesia, allodynia), vasomotor (temperature asymmetry, skin color changes), sudomotor/edema (edema, sweating asymmetry), and motor/trophic (decreased range of motion, tremors, dystonia, changes in hair/nail growth). Additionally, at least one sign in two or more of these categories must be observed on examination. Initial management included nonsteroidal anti-inflammatory drugs (NSAIDs), gabapentinoids, and physical therapy, with minimal symptom relief.

Symptoms and Signs of CRPS
CRPS is characterized by a constellation of sensory, autonomic, motor, and trophic changes that typically affect an extremity. The primary symptom is intense, disproportionate pain, often described as burning, stabbing, or throbbing. This pain is accompanied by hyperalgesia (increased sensitivity to pain) and allodynia (pain elicited by non-painful stimuli such as light touch). Autonomic dysfunction manifests as abnormal skin color changes, temperature asymmetry, and excessive sweating in the affected limb. Edema and swelling may also be present. Motor disturbances include weakness, tremors, dystonia, and impaired coordination. Trophic changes, including alterations in hair growth, nail texture, and skin atrophy, further contribute to the clinical picture. These symptoms often progress in stages, with early intervention being crucial for a better prognosis.

Due to inadequate response to conventional therapy, the patient was started on LDN at a dose of 4.5 mg once a day. Within six weeks of initiating LDN, the patient reported a marked reduction in pain intensity, improved mobility, and diminished sensory abnormalities. By three months, her functional status had significantly improved, and pain levels had decreased by more than 50%. No adverse effects were reported.

Central Sensitization and CRPS
CRPS is strongly linked to Central Sensitization, a process in which the central nervous system becomes hyperresponsive to stimuli following an initial injury. This heightened response is driven by increased excitability of neurons in the dorsal horn, persistent microglial activation, and altered pain processing pathways. Central sensitization leads to exaggerated pain perception, hyperalgesia, and allodynia, contributing to the chronic and often refractory nature of CRPS. Given its role in modulating neuroinflammation and glial cell activation, LDN has been proposed as a promising therapeutic option for conditions characterized by central sensitization, including CRPS .

Glial Cell Activation and Pain Modulation
Glial cells, including microglia and astrocytes, play a crucial role in the development and maintenance of central sensitization. Following an injury or prolonged pain stimulus, microglia become activated and release pro-inflammatory cytokines such as interleukin-1β (IL-1β), interleukin-6 (IL-6), and tumor necrosis factor-alpha (TNF-α). These inflammatory mediators enhance synaptic transmission, increase neuronal excitability, and decrease endogenous pain inhibition, leading to sustained pain hypersensitivity. Additionally, astrocytes contribute to neuroinflammation by releasing glutamate and other excitatory neurotransmitters that exacerbate pain signaling. By modulating microglial activation and reducing neuroinflammatory cascades, LDN may help restore normal pain processing and mitigate the symptoms of CRPS.

Toll-Like Receptors and Pain Modulation
LDN has been shown to modulate the activity of toll-like receptors (TLRs), particularly TLR4, which is predominantly expressed in microglia. TLR4 activation plays a key role in the propagation of

neuroinflammation and chronic pain by triggering the release of pro-inflammatory cytokines and excitatory neurotransmitters. By acting as a partial antagonist to TLR4, LDN reduces the inflammatory signaling that contributes to central sensitization and persistent pain. This effect helps to decrease neuronal excitability and ultimately leads to improved pain modulation, making LDN a promising therapeutic option for CRPS and other chronic pain disorders.

Opioid Growth Factor and Pain Modulation
LDN has also been shown to influence the opioid growth factor (OGF) pathway, which plays a critical role in pain modulation and immune regulation. OGF, also known as met-enkephalin, binds to the opioid growth factor receptor (OGFr) and regulates cell proliferation and immune function. LDN temporarily blocks the OGF-OGFr interaction, leading to a compensatory increase in endogenous OGF production and receptor sensitivity. This enhanced OGF activity helps to modulate pain perception, reduce neuroinflammation, and promote tissue repair, further contributing to LDN's therapeutic effects in CRPS and other chronic pain conditions.

Discussion
LDN is increasingly recognized for its potential benefits in chronic pain conditions, likely mediated through its effects on microglial modulation and opioid receptor antagonism. LDN exerts its analgesic effects through several mechanisms. First, it temporarily blocks opioid receptors, leading to a compensatory upregulation of endogenous opioid production, enhancing natural pain relief. Additionally, LDN modulates microglial activity, reducing the release of pro-inflammatory cytokines such as IL-1β, IL-6, and TNF-α. By dampening neuroinflammation, LDN helps decrease neuronal excitability and interrupt the cycle of central sensitization. Furthermore, LDN has been shown to promote neuroprotection

and enhance mitochondrial function, potentially contributing to its efficacy in CRPS and other chronic pain syndromes.

Conclusion
This case highlights the potential efficacy and safety of LDN in managing CRPS. Given its favorable safety profile and promising outcomes, LDN may represent an important addition to the therapeutic armamentarium for CRPS. Future clinical trials are warranted to establish standardized treatment protocols.

Introduction to LDN as an Adjunct to Psychotherapy

Galyn Forster, MS

The purpose of this introduction is to orient the reader to how the author and others are using low dose naltrexone (LDN) as an adjunctive to psychotherapy. We will look at how our mental health (MH) treatment strategy differs from how LDN is typically used to treat other medical conditions. I will also briefly explore research about the opioid system that may help explain the clinical results we have observed. The following case studies involve clients dealing with traumatic stress, dissociation, and pain and require some clarification of terms, but it is outside the scope of this introduction to do more than touch on the underlying bio-psychological mechanisms relevant for understanding how LDN and other opioid antagonists provide therapeutic benefits.

For an introduction to trauma, post-traumatic stress disorder (PTSD), complex-PTSD (CPTSD) and dissociative disorders, and treatment with LDN the reader is referred to The LDN Book Volume Two, chapters 9 and 10 (Lanius, Forster, and Pape, in Elsegood, 2020) (see also Lanius, U., et al., 2014; Escamilla, et al., 2023). My primary goal is to offer a roadmap of the underlying biochemistry to explain how opioid antagonists such as LDN appear to moderate/suppress protective-sympathetic activation (fight, flight and freeze), as well as disrupting habitual and addictive behavior in favor of goal driven behavior.

Emotions, Defensive Responses

Defensive responses are hardwired, physically-based emotional responses to threat designed to maximize survival (Panksepp and Biven, 2012). "Fight and Flight" are the defensive responses that most commonly come to mind when one thinks of PTSD and responses to threat in general, but there are others. Panksepp identifies the following hardwired mammalian defensive emotions: SEEKING protection, RAGE or Fight, FEAR or Flight, as well as PANIC or immobilization. These defensive responses commonly occur in a hierarchical fashion, and are expressed based on individual differences, including genetic predisposition, the nature of the threat, as well as the context of the threat.

Dissociative Disorders Endogenous Opioids, Stress
Dissociative symptoms vary by type and severity. They commonly affect the person's sense of identity, memory, and consciousness, as well as self-awareness and awareness of one's surroundings, and may include the following: depersonalization, derealization, amnesia, significant memory lapses, affect dysregulation, unexpected mood shifts, depression and/or anxiety, cognitive (thought-related) problem, vulnerability to pain disorders.

Dissociation is mediated, at least in part, by endogenous opioids (Scaer, 2001; Schore, 2001), which may account for dissociative phenomena like numbing, confusion, cognitive impairment, and amnesia (Bremner and Brett, 1997). Decades of research suggest that exposure to overwhelming trauma often results in a sustained period of analgesia. Soldiers wounded in battle frequently require much lower doses of morphine than the doses needed by patients injured in non-combat contexts (Beecher, 1946).

Treating PTSD, CPTSD, Dissociation and other MH Issues with LDN:

First-line treatments for PTSD include individual trauma-focused cognitive behavioral therapy (TF-CBT) and eye movement desensitization and reprocessing therapy (EMDR), which have been demonstrated to be effective for reducing clinician-rated PTSD symptoms (Ostacher and Cifu, 2018). Pharmacological treatments are effective to a lesser degree and considered second-line treatments for managing PTSD symptoms (Coventry, et al., 2020).

Complex PTSD (CPTSD) has recently been identified as a distinct variation of PTSD in the 11th edition of the International Statistical Classification of Diseases (ICD-11). In addition to the core PTSD symptoms, it includes symptoms associated with disturbances of self-organization, affect dysregulation, negative self-concept, and interpersonal problems. The disorder has a 1-8% population prevalence and up to 50% prevalence in mental health facilities." (Maercker, et al., 2022).

In the author's experience, LDN has shown beneficial effects on PTSD, CPTSD, and other MH issues, particularly when there are significant dissociative symptoms, and it appears to have clear benefits as an adjunctive to psychotherapy beyond that offered by conventional pharmacological interventions, with minimal side effects. Psychoactive pharmaceuticals frequently blunt emotional experience or induce dissociative-like states, whereas LDN and other opioid antagonists appear to disrupt dissociation and increase alertness, emotional experience, and present-time awareness.

Naltrexone Dosing
There are a limited number of studies focused on high-dose naltrexone treatment (50 mg - 400 mg a day) for dissociation and PTSD (see Escamilla, et al., 2023; Lanius, et al., 2018), but there are only two studies directly focused on LDN, both with promising results: a pilot trial focused on depression (Mischoulon, et al., 2017) and a study focused on treating dissociation and complex trauma with LDN (Pape and Wholer, 2015). With regard to naltrexone, a nonlinear dosage effect has been reported (e.g., Castellano and Puglisi-Allegra, 1982). That is, the magnitude of change does not correspond proportionally to dose size. At this time, there are no formally established dosing protocols for treating PTSD with LDN or with high naltrexone doses.

LDN MH Treatment is Tied to Multiple Mechanisms of Action
I believe the benefits from the use of multiple daily LDN doses are generated via four different biochemical mechanisms working synergistically.

The following is a proposed map of the neurobiological mechanisms by which LDN generates the positive treatment effects observed in my psychotherapy practice. Lacking direct testing on LDN, these observations are based on current research about the opioid system's contribution to habits and addictions, and to protective autonomic nervous system reactivity, the opioid system's contribution to the creation and expression of dissociative pathology, and the demonstrated ability of opioid antagonists to disrupt both protective autonomic system reactivity and dissociation.

I label regulatory/structural effects related to a single daily LDN dose as type 1a and 1b respectively. Effects resulting from multiple daily dosing tied to a small, constant serum blood level presence are labeled as type 2a and 2b. The latter appear to disrupt protective autonomic reactivity and habitual and addictive behavioral patterns.

Type 1 Effects
Two persistent regulatory alterations to neurological status: Type 1a enhanced immune system functioning, and Type 1b upregulation of opioid receptors and peptides

Type 1a Effects
A single daily LDN dose may facilitate regulating effects on the opioid system and the larger immune system, enhancing the healthy functioning of these mutually regulating systems. The enhanced functionality may reduce the stress load, resulting in improved physical and psychological health. This functional improvement is described by clinicians and researchers familiar with LDN as a 'stimulation-regulation' effect.

As an opioid antagonist, LDN alters opioid system functioning, triggering a subtle but powerful rebound effect that increases opioid receptor and neurotransmitter production, with synergistic improvements in dopamine function (Mischoulon et al., 2017) due to the fact that the dopamine and opioid systems mutually regulate one another. It also has an antagonizing (moderating) effect on certain toll-like receptors (TLRs), including TLR-4 which is responsible for activation of microglia and other components of the immune system that contribute to inflammation and to autoimmunity. Its antagonizing of TLR-4 receptors on microglia reduces excess inflammation. (Kučić, et al., 2021; Younger, et al., 2014) This is important because excess inflammation is a significant component of mental and somatic health pathology (Miller et al., 2018). These LDN-facilitated improvements to the opioid and immune systems result in improved health overall. For some patients, these effects alone may be adequate to produce antidepressant and anti-anxiety effects (Shukhman and Shukhman, 2016).

Type 1b Effects
There is a second type 1 effect that benefits survivors of early trauma and neglect. These individuals are more vulnerable to experiencing multiple forms of dissociation. Experience of childhood neglect and abuse often results in a physiology adapted for survival in a threatening, dangerous world (Teicher and Samson, 2016), but not optimal for living in a safe, supportive environment. This adaptation includes reductions in the baseline expression/production of opioid receptors and neurotransmitters in specific areas of the brain. These changes can then compromise one's ability to regulate strong emotional states (Schore, 2001).

In response to perceived threats, the truncated opioid systems of these abuse survivors experience rapid saturation by endogenous opioids (EOs), triggering a premature default to protective-sympathetic responses (fight, flight, freeze). If the perception of threat persists and the attempt to mount a sympathetic defense is ineffective, they may be more vulnerable to experiencing parasympathetic collapse, a state mediated by a massive flood of opioids (Lanius and Corrigan, 2014; Roelofs, 2017).

By increasing production of both EO receptors and neurotransmitters, LDN may slow opioid system flooding of available receptors, thereby blocking exaggerated perceptions of danger and threat. When this bio-psychological protective reaction, experienced as dissociation, is blocked, the individual experiences increased response flexibility. Opioid receptor sensitivity, altered by the effect of an opioid antagonist, could also contribute to this effect.

Dissociation

Since the reduction of dissociative symptoms associated with multiple daytime dosing is a primary benefit of what I refer to as Type 2 effects, a brief introduction to how I think about dissociation is in order; partly because I use the term more broadly than some experts do. In addition to using the term to describe symptoms of depersonalization, derealization, numbing, dysphoria, as well as flashback-type experiences, I also employ it to describe more subtle trauma-memory shaped alterations to perceptions, emotional states, and consciousness.

In the trauma treatment and research field, there have been many disagreements about the causes and essential characteristics of what gets labeled dissociation. The issue is complicated by the fact that the word 'dissociation' is used to describe hard-wired biologically based responses to threatening events, and these same responses generate an array of bio-psycho-behavioral symptoms also labeled 'dissociation.' Automatic/trance-like mental states often accompany addictive and habitual behaviors and also have a dissociative quality to them (also with opioid system involvement). Additionally, there are normative, non-pathological forms of dissociation, such as daydreaming or driving in a trance-like state.

1.) When applied to traumatic stress disorders, the word 'dissociation' describes a biologically based alteration (both conditioned and unconditioned) of function and perception associated with reactions to threatening experiences.

2.) In reaction to experiences of extreme stress or threats to survival, various types of dissociative symptoms emerge. Sometimes, these symptoms include explicit narrative memory; more often than not, there is no story, just implicit emotional conditioning. When a traumatic memory is activated—whether explicit or implicit— the organism reproduces an approximation of the neurophysiology associated with the original experience, the event is re-experienced rather than merely recollected.

A prominent example of dissociation is when the flashback of a traumatic event eclipses present-time perceptions of reality; the person is caught up in the past trauma as if they are reliving it. Less obvious, but also dissociative, is the activation of fear conditioning absent explicit narrative memory, distorting present-time perceptions, feelings and cognitions. This could be triggered by something as simple as a smell, a word, a tone of voice, or anything associated with a past stressor or threat.

At its root, the word 'dissociation' means disconnection. The individual's awareness is no longer engaged solely with the present place, person, or time. With pathological dissociation, there is also an "associating" component, linking the individual's perceptions with implicit emotional memory from past trauma. This emotional reaction, divorced from narrative memory, is then at risk to loop over and over.

Endogenous opioids (EO) are actively involved in the defensive-response cascade — both sympathetic and parasympathetic — and play a central role in the biochemistry underlying dissociative reactivity. Different dissociative symptoms emerge depending on how far along the defensive cascade the individual originally progressed. For example, sympathetic activation expressed as rage vs. the extreme confusion and physical collapse accompanying a parasympathetic defeat response: opposite ends of a continuum.

As the defensive cascade progresses—from an active sympathetic response to the ultimate, passive parasympathetic collapse—access to higher-order brain functioning progressively diminishes (Kozlowska, et al., 2015; Roelofs, and Dayan, 2022; Lanius, et al., 2018; Lanius, 2014). The derivative dissociative symptoms may or may not mirror the original defensive cascade.

Type 2 Effects

LDN appears to alter present-time EO contributions to the defensive cascade as well as altering underlying EO contributions to habitual and addictive behavior patterns. These alterations disrupt associated dissociative phenomena. Whether the issue relates to protective autonomic reactivity or to habitual behaviors, LDN's disruptive effect depends on maintaining an adequate naltrexone serum-blood-level presence. A single high dose of naltrexone accomplishes this, but due to naltrexone's short half-life (approximately 4 hours), LDN requires multiple doses to maintain effectiveness.

Type 2a effects: EOs contribute to many different dissociative symptoms, generated by the analgesia associated with both sympathetic and parasympathetic protective reactions. The contribution of EOs to protective-sympathetic activation (prSa—fight-flight-freeze) is often overlooked. First, because endocannabinoids appear to be the primary source of analgesia during the flight-fight-freeze response, and second, because EO contribution to prSa is relatively small. By comparison, EOs play a major role in parasympathetic defeat and collapse states (Lannius, et al., 2018). The sympathetic and parasympathetic systems are often portrayed as a binary as if they work in opposition to one another, but homeostasis requires that both be present, with one or the other being dominant.

Whether attributable to subtle prPSa or intrinsic to prSa, EOs appear to play a role in prSa and related analgesia, as demonstrated by the opioid antagonist naloxone's ability to disrupt prSa (Binder, et al., 2004; Fechir, et al., 2012; Lanius, et al., 2014)).

In addition to fight or flight, the prSa includes a freeze response - a temporary parasympathetic brake on the fight-flight response (Roelofs and Dayan, 2022). This is distinct from parasympathetic collapse. Freeze is thought to have evolved as a strategy to avoid detection by predators. An example in nature of this prSa is a deer automatically freezing when it perceives a threat but immediately fleeing when the coast is clear. An opossum unable to escape a threat provides an example of tonic immobility or parasympathetic collapse: it roles over and in a state of tonic immobility, displaying multiple symptoms that mimic death, becomes limp thus, the term "playing possum." It is common for rape survivors to report being mentally alert, in a state of prSa, wanting to mount an active defense but being physically frozen, unable to move. Superficially, the sympathetic freeze response could be mistaken for parasympathetic collapse, but the physiology is very different.

The analgesia associated with prSa appears to support mounting an effective defense by overriding distractions from the pain of an injury. Endocannabinoids are the primary source of prSa-activated analgesia, but opioids are also involved. Naltrexone has been shown to block anger-induced analgesia before the induction of pain, demonstrating opioid involvement (Burns, et al., 2009). The same endocannabinoid and opioid activity that produces analgesia in prSa also disrupts normal communication between lower and higher brain structures, resulting in dissociative phenomena associated with high arousal (Bracken, et al., 2008; Johnson, et al., 2022). Examples of dissociation associated with the prSa part of the protective cascade might include fleeing an uncomfortable conversation or responding with disproportionate anger, excessive defensiveness in a domestic conflict, or fighting in a blackout rage.

Some forms of non-suicidal self harm appear to be a behavioral strategy in which EO-mediated analgesia disrupts higher-order brain functioning, triggering a dissociative reaction to regulate highly aversive emotional states (Johnson, et al., 2022; Fechir, et al., 2012).

When treating complex PTSD and other trauma-related conditions, a single high dose of naltrexone will block dissociation. This effect appears to depend on maintaining an adequate serum blood level presence of naltrexone. Due to naltrexone's short serum blood half-life of 4-6 hours, treating MH issues with LDN appears to require 2-4 daily doses to maintain an adequate naltrexone presence. High doses of naltrexone antagonize a high percentage of opioid receptors, in contrast, multiple LDN doses appear to maintain a constant partial opioid blockade and apparently do so without compromising immune system benefits lost at high naltrexone doses.

Type 2b effects extend to substance-based and behavioral addictions and habits. In addition to directly altering the chemistry underlying chemical addictions, it appears that LDN, like higher doses of naltrexone, alters the neurobiology of the automatic, trance-like mental state one enters when engaging in addictive or habitual behavior (patterns based on repeated conditioning). Neurochemically, this effect appears to involve the switching of dominance between the dopamine and opioid systems expressed in addiction and habit-driven vs. reward-driven behaviors (Voon, et al., 2020; See also, Wardle, et al., 2016). Spencer and colleagues (2023) recently demonstrated that naltrexone influences this shift, 'not from directly modifying the endogenous opioid system's modulation of dopamine release as the mechanism reducing attentional bias to conditioned cues'. Instead, naltrexone's effect was found to be due primarily to an increase in top-down control of attention (increased activation of the putamen and pallidum). Bottom line: the power of conditioning associated with addictions, as well as habits, is weakened in favor of present time, mindful, responsiveness to actual rewards and risks, immediate and future. Multiple doses of LDN appear to prioritize current rewards over past conditioning.

While there is a great deal of overlap, the biologies of habit and addiction, of protective autonomic activation, and dissociation are distinct processes, often intimately entangled but sometimes less so.

Summary
Type 1 effects are generated by a single daily dose: Type 1a effects improve immune system regulation, and type 1b effects enhance opioid system functioning due to the up-regulation of opioid receptors and opioid neurotransmitters, weakening the proclivity to dissociate. Together, these regulation-based improvements promote somatic health and emotional well-being.

Type 2 effects are generated by 2-4 daily doses: Type 2a effects suppress present-time protective autonomic reactivity and dissociation. Type 2b effects disrupt addiction and habit-driven behaviors. The majority of MH symptoms appear to respond most robustly to an LDN treatment regimen of multiple daily doses.

While the constant partial opioid blockade associated with multiple daily LDN dosing is counter-indicated when treating some somatic disorders, I have not observed compromises of immune system benefits in the more than 100 MH cases with which I have worked. Typically there was evidence of improved immune system function, even when not originally identified as a treatment target (e.g., reduced pain or asthma symptoms).

Pain, Dissociation and Opioid Antagonists
The current understanding of pain includes not only injury to tissue or a disease state but also the threat of injury (Butler and Moseley, 2003).

While not considered an emotion, the perception of pain typically triggers survival-based emotional reactions. The perception of threat plays an active role in whether or not something is interpreted as pain and in the perceived magnitude of the pain. The brain is centrally involved in the generation of and perception of pain. Like other threatening and stressful experiences, pain is remembered, both as part of narrative memories and in the form of implicit memory. Like other traumatic memories and conditioned associations, these pain memories can also be associatively triggered. It is commonly reported by EMDR Therapy clinicians that during processing clients will report spontaneously re-experiencing somatic pain associated with traumatic memories, e.g., bodily feeling somatic pain from a past trauma. Headaches are a common example; the pain arises out of nowhere during processing and, just as quickly, disappears as the client recognizes present time safety.

It follows that just as implicit memory of past trauma can exaggerate the feelings of threat and danger in social interactions, so also, implicit memory of a previous painful experience can merge with and exaggerate the perception of a current painful experience. Informed by past experience, the brain may generate a pain response based more on the memory of past painful experiences rather than just what is happening in the body. This can affect the perception of both acute and persistent/chronic pain (pain without an identifiable acute cause). While multiple potential nervous system disorders are contributing to persistent pain, dissociative memory likely plays a role in many cases.

While there is evidence that single LDN doses are more effective treating chronic pain than high doses of naltrexone (Kim and Fishman, 2020), to my knowledge there are no controlled studies exploring whether multiple daily doses compromise or improve-on the benefits of a single LDN dose. Nevertheless, in my experience with MII cases, as reported in the following case studies, both acute and chronic pain appear to respond well to a regimen of multiple LDN doses.

The majority of what I have identified as Type 1 and Type 2 LDN treatment effects easily transfer to the treatment of pain without requiring significant modification.

Clinical Considerations

Psycho-education is important when working with this population. LDN's reduction of dissociation sets some patients up to initially mistake an increased experience of their own emotions as a negative side effect. Without the buffer of dissociation, feeling affects more distinctly and particularly experiencing positive affect can feel overwhelming and, at first, may be experienced as aversive.

LDN treatment of MH patients should be initiated gradually, especially if the patient is medically fragile or highly dissociative. Otherwise, if they are medically stable, once they demonstrate LDN is well-tolerated, dose levels can be increased rapidly, often reaching the target dose in a matter of days, rarely requiring longer than a couple of weeks. 0.06 mg/kg body weight taken 2-4 times daily is a good guide for setting an initial target dose, but this should be modified based on the patient's response. I always advise that they begin treatment with a single dose, no more than half the target dose, taken in the morning to avoid sleep disruption, on the off-chance they might be among the 10 percent for which it disrupts falling asleep if taken close to bedtime. Once the single target dose is established it is time to identify how many doses best serve the patient. Periodically, the clinician should monitor compliance and adjust the daily regimen if needed. Because the effects can be subtle (and there are no withdrawals if they stop LDN), it is common for patients to underestimate the benefits they are getting from LDN. Chapter 10 of The LDN Book Volume 2 includes more in-depth coverage of clinical considerations for treating MH conditions with LDN (Lanus and Forster, 2020).

Mental Health and Somatic Disorders

Complex Trauma and Autoimmune Disorders

Galyn Forster, MS

Abstract

This case explores low dose naltrexone (LDN) as an adjunctive to psychotherapy in the treatment of a forty-year-old female, a trauma survivor with comorbid rheumatoid arthritis (RA), lupus, and chronic pain, all of which were better managed with LDN than with conventional treatments. Interestingly, LDN appears to have served as an augmentation agent for a previously ineffective steroidal therapeutic for treatment of RA. Complications from extreme sleep deprivation had to be resolved before she obtained the maximum benefit that comes from multiple daytime doses of LDN.

Introduction

This case illustrates the complexities that can arise using multiple daytime LDN doses as an adjunctive to psychotherapy when the patient is also navigating pain and symptoms from RA, Lupus, and thyroiditis. Initially, a solitary evening dose significantly reduced RA symptoms and pain, as well as post-traumatic stress disorder (PTSD) symptoms of emotional reactivity and dissociation, before she was able to tolerate multiple daytime dosing. Eventually, she was able to tolerate a multiple daily dosing protocol, though initially, sleep deprivation prevented or complicated daytime LDN dosing. However, after this was resolved, LDN further improved each disordered state.

A history of early childhood exposure to trauma and neglect usually correlates with positive outcomes from adjunctive LDN treatment with psychotherapy. This is due, at least in part, to the fact that childhood exposure to neglect and trauma remodels the young brain to better equip it for survival in a hostile world. The endogenous opioid system is modified, permanently reducing the abundance of opioid receptors in regions of the brain involved in survival and threat detection. (Schore, 2001; Lanius, et al., 2014; Lanius and Forster, 2020). Her symptoms of dissociation, hypervigilance, and anger issues suggested this client would be a good candidate for LDN.

LDN therapy for trauma and dissociative disorders is supported by anecdotal evidence and a limited body of research focused on opioid antagonist treatment of trauma and dissociation. The current research provides evidence that opioid antagonists can disrupt protective dissociative responses commonly associated with trauma and dissociative disorders. (Pape and Wöller, 2015). In their systemic literature review, "Treatment of dissociative symptoms with opioid antagonists", Escamilla and colleagues conclude, "Opioid antagonists (particularly naltrexone) are promising candidates for the treatment of dissociative symptoms". (Escamilla, et al., 2023; Lanius, et al., 2014; Timäus, et al., 2023). See the introduction for a more in-depth discussion of this topic.

I find that LDN significantly improves moment-to-moment emotional regulation for most trauma survivors, quality of life, and treatment outcomes. It also has the potential to better manage pain and other symptoms from RA, lupus, and thyroiditis.

Rheumatoid arthritis (RA) and lupus are both autoimmune diseases, but they are distinct from one another. Lupus is not arthritis but can have arthritis as a symptom. Drug-induced lupus is a rare autoimmune disorder triggered by chronic use of certain medications. RA primarily affects the joints, while lupus can affect any body part, including the joints, skin, kidneys, brain, and other organs. Women are 2 to 3 times more likely than men to have RA and up to 9 times more likely to have Lupus.

Concerning the potential to reduce symptoms from RA and lupus, multiple studies have characterized LDN as a promising and safe therapy for pain management, including from rheumatic diseases. (Dara,et al., 2023; de Carvalho and Skare, 2023). A controlled before-after study grounded on the Norwegian Prescription Database (NorPD) compared prescriptions to RA patients one year before and one year after starting LDN and found a reduction in the use of NSAIDs, opioids, and disease-modifying antirheumatic drugs (DMARDs) such as methotrexate and anti-TNF-alpha drugs. (Raknes and Småbrekke, 2019).

Patient Description and Diagnoses

A 40-year-old mother of a four-year-old and triplets, being treated for complex PTSD and pain, in long-term recovery from alcohol and behavioral addictions. She was diagnosed with rheumatoid arthritis (RA) at the age of 15, and at 30 with drug-induced lupus. She was also being treated for Hashimoto's thyroiditis, for which she was taking 175 mcg of levothyroxine. RA and lupus caused body aches, joint pain, compromised her flexibility and range of motion, and periodically flares left her bedridden for days on end. For self-care, she kept a healthy diet, exercised daily, and walked for up to an hour most days. As if caring for triplets and a sibling four years older was not exercise enough.

In the distant past, her RA flares were treated with prednisone and infliximab (Remicade) infusions. More recently, RA flares were treated with standard of care therapeutics, including methylprednisolone (32 mg dose packs or daily doses of 50 mg) for up to six days at a time. These medications were only marginally effective and, due to unpleasant side effects, she only used them two or three times a year, when RA flares were unmanageable. When she began treatment with me, she was primarily using nonsteroidal anti-inflammatory drugs (NSAIDs) and acctaminophen for pain relief.

Presenting Problems

Mental Health: After a five-year break from psychotherapy, she resumed therapy following the trauma-filled experience of giving birth to triplets; her life and that of one of the triplets had been endangered while giving birth and immediately following the birth. This trauma was magnified by her own, unresolved birth-trauma and subsequent lack of nurture from a critical, depressed mother.

Her trauma score of 59, using the PCL-5, a PTSD self-report inventory, placed her in the severe range for PTSD (see below for more details). Her family of origin-based dismissing-avoidant attachment style often resulted in her withholding and withdrawing when there were relationship challenges with her husband. While committed to one another and their family, the task of caring for four young children exhausted both parents and strained their relationship. One of her attachment-related trauma symptoms was a phobia of shared positive-affect (mistrusting and finding positive feelings uncomfortable) which presents distinct challenges for building and maintaining intimate relationships.

In the past, she learned to constructively channel stress-triggered dissociation into a partially numbed-out state, void of virtually all emotion. In this state she did not feel resentment or rage, she was calm and could "handle anything that happened, and do what I need to do", instead of an older pattern of "making things worse". Dissociating this way began with "a warm feeling flowing through me as if someone inserted an IV with heroin." She was unavailable for emotional connection but was still able to get things done. Biochemically, she likely experienced a moderate flood of endogenous opioids (and endocannabinoids), not unlike a small dose of morphine, but not so great that she was incapacitated into euphoria or a parasympathetic collapse state. Her description of "a warm feeling" suggests a greater endogenous opioid dose than typically accompanies a protective-sympathetic, fight-flight, response, which numbs the awareness of pain until after the threat is addressed. (See this chapter's introduction.)

RA, Lupus, Hashimoto's, and Pain: She was in constant pain from RA and lupus; physical movement was painful and difficult. Before LDN therapy, her pain baseline was 2 or 3 (on a 0 to 10 scale) but would spike much higher with stress and exhaustion. She mostly ignored lower levels of pain, focusing on the work at hand. Symptoms of lupus included muscle aches and pain, painful breathing, anemia, fatigue, fever, mouth dryness and ulcers of the mouth, rashes, butterfly rash on her face, hair loss, joint stiffness and flares, Raynaud's syndrome, sensitivity to light and swelling with water retention. Hashimoto's thyroiditis added to fatigue and contributed to hair loss. To cope with the constant discomfort, she sometimes dissociated, finding a numbed escape; however, at other times, this led to a cold, emotionless rage.

Treatment Plan and Implementation

A month after resuming psychotherapy, she began LDN treatment as an adjunctive to psychotherapy to help manage emotional reactivity, reduce dissociation, and better tolerate the process of facing trauma during therapy. In addition, it was hoped LDN would reduce pain and stabilize lupus and RA symptoms. The long-term treatment plan for LDN was for her to eventually be taking two to three doses daily using the formula of 0.06 mg/kg of body weight. To allow the patient's body to adjust gradually and to avoid side effects, they initiate LDN treatment with half the target dose, or even less if they are particularly sensitive. The dose is then increased as quickly as they can comfortably tolerate.

She initiated LDN treatment with 1.5 mg the first week and increased it to 2 mg the second week. Because this client was being treated for autoimmune disorders, as well as for PTSD, she increased her dose more slowly than is required for most mental health patients. They often titrate up to their target dose, b.i.d. or t.i.d., in one or two weeks. Since there were no negative side effects, she increased the dose weekly by 1.5 mg until reaching her target of 4.5 mg. She found 3 mg more comfortable so she reduced back to that dose.

To rule out the possibility LDN might give her energy and interfere with sleep, she took her first dose in the morning, but the opposite happened, it made her sleepy. She shifted to taking LDN in the evening before going to bed; this reduced tension and improved sleep quality. The second week she reported that the day following a 2 mg evening dose, she had less pain and "it was not as difficult to do things." In addition, instead of feeling pain "all over", the reduced pain localized in her hips, hands, and shoulder. If she missed her evening dose, she noticed an immediate increase in pain the next day. The localized pain may have been acute pain related to inflammation, reduced but not fully resolved, and the greater generalized pain may have been an expression of dissociation based chronic pain, a somatic memory.

The unusual side effect of daytime sleepiness is interesting. I believe it occurred because, as a mother of a 4-year-old and 4-month-old triplets, she was exhausted and constantly sleep deprived, by dissociating/compartmentalizing the awareness of the need for sleep, she was able to focus on the demands of being a mother. Motherhood had priority over rest.

Taking LDN during the day appeared to disrupt her automatic, habit-based dissociating of the awareness of feeling tired and sleepy. This involves increasing sympathetic tone, similar to what we experience in the fight-flight response to a threat, but probably on a smaller scale, and without the threat component. Opioids and dopamine are both centrally involved in determining whether behaviors will be of a habitual nature (automatic) or determined by the organism's immediate needs. (Sharp, et al., 2015; Majuri, et al.,

2016; Voon et al, 2020; Mikus, et al., 2022). LDN and other opioid antagonists, alter this dopamine-opioid balance so that goal-directed behavior is prioritized over habit and addiction-based behavior (learned patterns). In her case, dissociating awareness of exhaustion would fall in the category of habit, while responding to exhaustion would be an example of being goal driven at a basic biological level.

One of my first clients to use LDN was highly anxious and always sleep-deprived, initially she responded to LDN as if it was a sedative: twenty minutes after taking her first dose she was sleeping soundly and out for the night. Two weeks later, having adjusted to the medication and no longer being sleep deprived, LDN lost the dramatic sedating effect but continued to improve sleep quality by reducing fear and hypervigilance.

The second week after raising the dose to 2 mg, dissociating less, she noticed she was feeling all her emotions more distinctly and found navigating this new awareness confusing. Feeling feelings was unfamiliar, and while some were enjoyable, other parts were very uncomfortable. She reported it felt right to be more in touch with her feelings and that she wanted to experience feelings more fully, "but it seemed complicated and challenging to have them." This is an example of affect phobia, shaped by early attachment trauma, causing her to feel uncomfortable with any intense feeling, positive or negative; virtually all emotions caused some level of discomfort. In the past, these feelings would have been automatically dissociated, "It was like something in me just knew it was important to not feel good." However, with LDN she is gaining the ability to experience a multitude of feelings that would have been dissociated away.

Soon after this expanding of her emotional awareness, she had an uncharacteristically intense rage episode focused on her husband and the world, lasting about two days before spontaneously resolving. Learning to navigate previously dissociated feelings was uncomfortable and a lot of work. After about six months, feeling feelings became her new normal, and she came to appreciate having fuller access to her emotions. With LDN on board, it was easier to receive kindness and take in the good feelings of her husband and others.

The third week of taking LDN, she raised the dose from 2 mg to 3 mg and reported additional relief from RA-related pain, and movement was more fluid. Dreams were more intense though not bad (a common LDN side effect). Some clients taking LDN to address mental health issues will not experience a noticeable reduction of symptoms until after reaching the 0.06 mg/kg/b/w dose ratio, but like her, others will notice benefits at half this ratio, and go on to realize additional benefits when the full dose is reached.

Seven weeks later, her next therapy session was focused on early attachment trauma that was expressed in a terrifying dream. At my suggestion, before doing EMDR trauma-processing, she took a fresh dose of LDN to moderate emotional flooding and dissociation. As we began EMDR processing of the traumatic dream, she reported feeling like she was having an RA flare and showed me that she could barely bend her fingers. We continued EMDR processing (by now LDN was entering her bloodstream and brain) and as the emotional charge of the trauma began to resolve, her fingers began to bend more easily. When EMDR processing was complete, as indicated by her felt sense that the event was in the past and she was safe and no longer alone, her previously stiff joints were working well with minimal pain. By reducing dissociation, LDN helped her find the courage to face her fear and stay present doing EMDR Therapy trauma processing. Doing this work appeared to reduce the stress that was contributing to an RA flare. At the same time, LDN's anti-inflammatory properties may have directly reduced the inflammation contributing to the RA flare.

Over the following two years, she fine-tuned her LDN dose regimen to more effectively meet her current needs. Three years after starting LDN, she regularly tolerates daytime doses and takes one or two extra doses when the stress load increases beyond normal. Knowing this, at a recent holiday gathering, typically highly stressful, she took an extra LDN dose during the day. As a result, she was "less on guard, not as resentful and was able to relax instead of worrying." She observed that, "I didn't notice it at the time but, reflecting later, felt more content and happier during the gathering."

LDN Treatment Outcomes

Psychotherapy: LDN helped accomplish multiple psychotherapy goals by disrupting PTSD-related dissociation and emotional flooding. During stressful family gatherings, instead of feeling overwhelmed and powerless, she was able to regulate her emotions with an increased sense of agency and control over her RA-caused physical reactivity. She observed that in the moment, it is easy to overlook the difference until later when she notices telling herself, "Oh, that wasn't so bad," in reaction to challenges that would have left her overwhelmed and upset.

At the start of her most recent course of therapy, her total score on the PTSD Checklist for the DSM-5 (PCL-5) was 58, placing her in the severe category (40 - 60) just below the extreme category (60 - 80). Four years later, after 45 psychotherapy sessions, including EMDR Therapy, often accompanied by a fresh dose of LDN, her PCL-5 score reduced to equal 12, placing her in the moderate category, suggesting PTSD is in remission.

LDN appears to have significantly reduced obsessive-compulsive thinking and behaviors. Hair tearing now only occurs when she is extremely fatigued and stressed. Obsessive rumination about shame, resentment, regret, and the safety of her children, instead of being a constant, has mostly disappeared.

Concerning LDN's effect on her ability to process intense trauma, she stated, "I believe LDN inhibited dissociation and allowed me to show up in therapy, prepared to drop into powerful processing with my emotions ready and authentic."

RA, Lupus, Thyroiditis and Pain: As expected, RA and lupus-related inflammation and pain significantly reduced after starting LDN therapy. Sleep duration and quality improved, which further supported somatic and psychological health.

When stressed beyond what she could have handled in the past, or when she could tell an RA flare was imminent, taking an extra 3 or 4 mg of LDN helped her cope emotionally, without compromising alertness. If an RA flare broke through, 2 or 3 extra LDN doses spaced out over the next 24 hours, drinking green juice, and recognizing she was safe and loved appeared to help quiet inflammation and put the flare behind her. When she feels an RA flare developing and she could not take extra time for bedrest, she would take an extra dose of LDN plus prednisone to quickly knock down the flare. Prednisone alone was ineffective at resolving RA flares until she began taking LDN.

Since starting LDN, flares occur far less frequently and are shorter in duration. She reported, "Before LDN therapy, I was in constant low-level pain and when a flare hit, I was bedridden for days or weeks with pain at level 10 (on a 0-10 scale), two or three times a year. Now I have a one-day flare every 2-3 years."

Since starting LDN, her levothyroxine dose has been reduced from 175 mcg to 125 mcg.

Multiple vs Single Dosing Regimen:
Unusual for most of my clients using LDN to treat mental health issues, this client was taking a single daily dose most days for the first two years rather than multiple doses. Initially, she reported that LDN made her sleepy when taking it during the day. But when she was dealing with the emotional challenge of a family visit, she regularly took a second dose to better control RA flares, without

triggering the sleepiness that day-time dosing normally caused her. The same was true for PMS symptoms. No longer being constantly sleep deprived, blocking dissociation with LDN during the day no longer causes/uncovers daytime drowsiness.

With LDN she benefits psychologically; it has helped her learn to tolerate feeling her feelings instead of dissociating them, and emotional trauma from her past gets triggered far less frequently. She thinks more clearly and feels less vulnerable. Nevertheless, she is sometimes reluctant to take LDN, knowing it will keep her from dissociating, numbing out and shutting off feelings, as she did in the past. This unconscious strategy of numbing-out in a dissociative state, in the past, helped her avoid dealing with uncomfortable emotions and be mentally tough. She could then just power through whatever hard task she was dealing with. However, as she has become healthier, she has grown more comfortable with her emotions and has come to value how they enrich her life.

Conclusion

This case demonstrates how a single daily LDN dose significantly reduced RA, lupus, and PTSD-related symptoms. When feeling excessive stress, taking LDN p.r.n. further improved her psychological functioning and helped her manage RA-related flares better than just a single evening dose of LDN.

Previously ineffective conventional therapeutics such as prednisone, when used as an adjunctive with LDN, gained in effectiveness, possibly due to LDN's anti-inflammatory effects and ability to moderate autoimmunity without compromising healthy immune system responses. LDN appears to have served as an augmentation agent for treatment of RA flares. Mischoulon and colleagues observed that LDN had the same potentiating effect when used with dopaminergic antidepressants for patients with breakthrough symptoms of major depression. (Mischoulon, et al., 2017). Lanius and Corrigan observe the same phenomenon in Neurobiology and Treatment of Traumatic Dissociation, with examples of LDN augmenting the effectiveness of anti-depressants, warfarin, and antipsychotic medications, sometimes requiring dosage reductions of those medications to avoid overdosing effects from the original medication. (Lanius, et al., 2014).

Predictably, daytime sleepiness resolved when she was no longer chronically sleep-deprived, then a protocol of multiple daily LDN doses resulted in additional psychological progress and further reduced pain, lupus, RA, and thyroiditis-related symptoms.

This case highlights the importance of fine-tuning LDN protocols to match the patient's emerging condition. Months after the sleepiness resolved, this patient had to be encouraged to experiment with consistent daytime dosing; otherwise, she might have settled for the valuable but limited benefit of a single nighttime dose. Morning, evening, and dosing when required, further reduced pain and other symptoms related to RA and PTSD.

Treatment Approaches for PTSD and Dissociation

Galyn Forster, MS

Abstract

This study examines the use of low dose naltrexone (LDN) as an adjunctive treatment to EMDR Therapy (EMDR) and talk therapy treatment of a client with post-traumatic stress disorder (PTSD) with dissociation and attention deficit hyperactivity disorder (ADHD). LDN treatment provided effective remediation of painful ear infections, a breast cyst, and an ovarian cyst, and it offered pain management for a badly injured knee before and after surgery, minimizing the need to use NSAIDs and other pain medication. Currently, there are no first-line pharmaceutical treatments for dissociation and PTSD, and the second-line pharmaceutical therapies are associated with negative side effects and less than robust outcomes.

While under-researched, opiate antagonists, such as naltrexone and LDN, offer an attractive alternative to conventional treatments; they directly moderate dissociative symptoms, and their toxicity and side effect profiles are comparatively low. In this case of a 48-year-old female, a regimen of multiple daily LDN doses focused on the treatment of mental health (MH) issues also effectively treated somatic issues. The case also illustrates the importance of carefully refining the dose regimen to accommodate the client's sensitivities and needs.

Introduction

According to the American Psychiatric Association Diagnostic and Statistical Manual of Mental Disorders, post-traumatic stress disorder (PTSD) is characterized by the appearance of debilitating symptoms that follow exposure to stressful traumatic events.

(American Psychiatric Association. 2022). Symptoms Include intrusive memories, avoidance, negative thoughts or mood, hyperarousal, possible cognitive impairment, difficulties with concentration, attention and memory, and a hyper-vigilance to threat. This study explores the utilization of LDN as an adjunctive treatment to EMDR Therapy and talk therapy for a 48-year-old woman with PTSD, dissociation, and painful somatic issues. We explore her psychiatric and medical history and describe the process of identifying an LDN dose regimen that accommodated her extreme sensitivity to medications. Her case illustrates how this MH protocol treats PTSD, dissociation and ADHD, while simultaneously treating painful somatic issues: chronic ear infections (otitis media), a micro cyst in a breast, and an ovarian cyst. LDN was also used as the primary pharmaceutical treatment for pain management pre- and post-surgery for a badly injured knee, reducing the need for other pain medications.

The use of LDN to address pain and immune system disorders is supported by a growing body of research. (Dara, et al., 2023; Rupp, et al., 2023; Toljan and Vrooman, 2018) As important neuromodulators, endogenous opioids play a critical role in the pathogenesis of multiple female reproductive disorders. Naltrexone and LDN have shown efficacy for the treatment of gynecological disorders. (Böttcher, et al., 2017; Torres-Reverón, et al., 2016; McKenzie-Brown, et al., 2021). Along with Metformin, LDN has been suggested as a first-line therapy, specifically, in hyperinsulinemic women with polycystic ovary syndrome.(Hadžiomerović-Pekić, et al., 2010).

A growing body of evidence supports the use of LDN for treatment of pain. (Praneet, et al., 2023; Rupp, et al., 2023; McKenzie-Brown, et al., 2023; Patten, et al., 2018; Marcus, et al., 2024).

Naltrexone and LDN therapy for trauma-based and dissociative disorders is supported by anecdotal evidence and a limited body of research. Though under-researched, the literature is supportive of using naltrexone and LDN to address dissociation and traumatic stress disorders. Endogenous opioids play an active role in the body's response to stress and threat. Opioid antagonists disrupt or moderate over-expression of protective responses which characterize trauma-based pathology. (Pape and Wöller, 2015). In their systemic literature review, Escamilla and colleagues conclude, "Opioid antagonists (particularly naltrexone) are promising candidates for the treatment of dissociative symptoms and showed a moderate – large effect size in reducing [dissociative] symptoms." (Escamilla, et al., 2023). Based on my clinical experience, I encouraged a trial of LDN as an adjunctive therapy to psychotherapy for this client.

Case History

Psychiatric and Somatic Symptoms: This is the case of a 48-year-old mother of two adult children, employed as a construction and maintenance worker. She was diagnosed with Complex PTSD with dissociation and also presented with symptoms of inattentive type ADHD. As a child, she experienced physical and sexual abuse by her alcoholic father who, according to her report, displayed symptoms suggestive of a dissociative disorder. As the oldest child, she learned to protect her younger siblings from their father's abuse but ended up dissociating when she could not protect herself. These early experiences provided challenges but, combined with an innate resilience and the loving care of her grandparents, she kept them from defining her as a person.

Symptoms of hypervigilance and anxiety would follow reminders of the trauma, sometimes triggering flashbacks to memories accompanied by a racing heart and shallow breathing. She avoided reminders of the past, felt cut off from others, was easily startled and suspicious of other people, and experienced blunted emotions and exaggerated guilt. Sleep quality was compromised by anxiety and intrusive dreams.

She suffered from chronic ear infections (otitis media), a micro cyst in one breast, and an ovarian cyst (previously requiring surgery), both of which were a daily source of pain.

Several months after resuming psychotherapy, she sustained a serious knee injury. Despite constant pain, she continued working for six months because her health insurance, ignoring her surgeon's expert opinion, delayed authorization of the necessary surgery.

I provided two episodes of psychotherapy separated by a break of ten years. Both treatment episodes were initiated after she had been hospitalized for psychiatric issues. The medical record identified PTSD as an issue but dissociative symptoms appear to have been minimized, leading to the interpretation of catatonia, confusion and depressive symptoms as evidence of psychosis. Although a reasonable initial assessment, her negative response to antipsychotics, history of dissociation and subsequent recovery suggest this diagnosis was in error.

After discontinuing her first course of therapy, she divorced her abusive husband and established a career as a construction and maintenance worker. For nine years she functioned well without psychiatric medication. Both times I worked with her she responded poorly to antipsychotics and had to dismiss unresponsive psychiatric providers before finding competent psychiatric care. After discontinuing the antipsychotics she stabilized psychologically and responded well to psychotherapy, focused on the treatment of trauma and dissociation.

Her second course of therapy was initiated three weeks after a psychiatric hospitalization caused by stress from months of harassment by her supervisor, ultimately forcing her to quit her primary employment. Two weeks later, she was found sitting in her car in the parking lot of her remaining place of employment (also not a safe environment) after her shift had started. She was non-responsive and appeared catatonic to people trying to assist her. She later described being able to hear and see the people wanting to help, but she was unable to communicate orally or execute physical movement. She distinctly recalled willing her hand to unlock the car door, but her hand would not move. She recalled that while being driven to the hospital by her son, she partially regained the ability to move again as she recognized feeling safe with him.

Diagnosis: At the hospital, her symptoms were misinterpreted as psychotic and she was diagnosed with "schizoaffective disorder, bipolar type, without good prognostic features." Review of her hospital records suggests her trauma history and the possibility of a dissociative diagnosis were minimized, resulting in a psychosis-related diagnosis, as had been the case when she was hospitalized ten years earlier. This may have been an example of clinicians diagnosing what they were most familiar with and for which they had a standard pharmaceutical treatment. Catatonia is often associated with psychotic disorders, but it has additional etiologies and is also associated with dissociative disorders. (Fink, M., et al., 2009; Longden, et al., 2020; Mahgoub, et al., 2024; Rosebush and Mazurek, 2009; Sarkar, et al., 2004).

She was treated with antipsychotics which were worse than ineffective: Olanzapine caused serious metabolic effects, the gaining of five pounds weekly (twice what is typical for olanzapine when rapid weight gain is an issue) until she discontinued its use. It also caused lethargy, compromising alertness and safety, for which she consumed excessive amounts of caffeine while at work. This, in turn, disrupted her sleep, further compromising her ability to function. An equally disturbing effect of olanzapine was 'feeling numb' to threat and danger as if she were immortal. She reported feeling no fear at the thought of walking into traffic or the idea of jumping off a three-story building (she categorically denied suicidal intent). When she complained about the excessive weight gain, instead of addressing her concerns, the psychiatrist informed her he was not her weight loss doctor.

In the past she had been prescribed multiple medications without benefit. Lorazepam made her "feel floaty and foggy minded". Risperidone caused lactation; quetiapine caused a rash and breathing issues; lamotrigine caused headaches and facial tremors; aripiprazole caused restless leg syndrome and akathisia, "feeling like she needed to move her body all the time".

To be clear, when a psychosis-related diagnosis is appropriate, antipsychotics are often necessary and beneficial, but they are not the standard of care for treating dissociation and trauma. There are no first-line pharmaceutical treatments for PTSD and dissociation. While not recognized as the standard of care or FDA-approved, research suggests dissociative pathology often responds positively to opioid antagonist treatments, including naltrexone and LDN. Clearly, more research is warranted. (Escamilla, et al., 2023; Timäus, et al., 2021; Lanius, et al., 2018). The first line of treatment for PTSD is trauma-focused psychotherapy (PE, CPT, and EMDR) and talk therapy for dissociation (specifically CBT, DT, and EMDR).

She resumed psychotherapy with me three weeks after being discharged from the hospital. A review of her hospital records, her dissociative history, and her narrative of events related to her recent hospitalization, supported my assessment that she was dealing with a PTSD-related dissociative episode rather than psychosis. Experiencing a catatonic-type state, while possibly suggestive of psychosis, may be caused by a variety of conditions, and also presents as a dissociative reaction to stress. In her case, extreme psychological stress, magnified by exhaustion and an allergic reaction to prednisone, appears to have resulted in tonic immobility and temporary paralysis. (Beutler, et al., 2022; Lanius, et al., 2018). The allergic reaction to prednisone was previously documented in her medical record. Still, it was overlooked by the physician treating her earaches and, later, by the two psychiatrists who dismissed her concerns about olanzapine's toxic side effects. They made it clear that, as the experts, they were uninterested in what she had to say, treating her as a willfully non-compliant patient wasting their time, even though she had dutifully taken every medication as prescribed until it began undermining her health, safety and ability to function.

Treatment Plan

Therapy focused on recent and past trauma, improving self-care, and helping her find supportive, competent psychiatric care. Two months after resuming counseling, at my suggestion, she decided to explore a trial of LDN to address PTSD and dissociation, as well as other medical conditions.

By the time LDN treatment was initiated, she was again working two eight-hour jobs. The supervisor's harassing behavior had been investigated, resulting in his termination and her reinstatement.

She started LDN with a dose slightly less than half of the 0.06 mg/kg/b/w ratio, which is typically helpful for treating PTSD and other MH conditions. She had a history of extreme sensitivity to medications, often requiring half of the standard dose. She also had allergic reactions to prednisone, morphine, codeine, and an anesthesia. At that time, she was physically and psychologically stable, so the more extreme caution necessary with physically fragile patients did not seem warranted when starting her LDN trial.

She began with 2 mg taken in the morning to avoid the risk of sleep disruption, on the chance she might be among the ten percent for whom LDN is energizing and prevents falling asleep for a few hours. It turned out she was among the ten percent, so she avoided late evening doses. Since she experienced no side effects during the first two or three days at 2 mg, she increased the size and frequency of her dose over the following two weeks to 5 mg in the morning and a second 3 mg dose at 4 pm, before starting her second eight-hour shift. This regimen worked well except that her focus and energy lagged the last two hours of her final shift, so further adjustments were made, including adding a 6 p.m. dose.

At the time this study was written, she was starting her day with 2 mg of LDN at 6 am to help her to wake up and focus. At 11:30 or noon she took 2 mg, and then a third 2 mg dose at 5:30 or 6:00 pm. The second and third doses helped maintain alertness and focus throughout the day. The last dose was particularly helpful for keeping energy levels up at the end of her long day. If she took it later than 5:30 or 6:00 pm, it prevented falling asleep promptly at midnight; if she took it two hours earlier, she was left dragging physically and the ADD symptoms returned before her second eight-hour shift was over. On days she had difficulty concentrating, or felt more anxious than normal, she increased the last dose to 4 mg.

Based on the formula of 0.06 mg/kg/b/w, this dose regimen was half what would typically be required for optimal effectiveness when treating PTSD and dissociative disorders, but it is what worked best for her.

Mental Health Benefits of Adding LDN: LDN appears to have significantly reduced PTSD symptoms. Before starting LDN treatment her total score on the DSM-5 self-report for PTSD (The PCL-5) was 65, placing her in the extreme category (60 - 80). LDN was added as an adjunctive to psychotherapy early in treatment. Two years later, when this case study was written, her PCL-5 score was 15, indicating her PTSD was in remission. During this time LDN helped disrupt dissociation and other PTSD symptoms, enhancing the progress that could be made in therapy. She continues to use it daily to help regulate emotions, reduce worry and ADHD symptoms, and treat somatic issues.

To be clear, much of the progress she made was the direct result of her psychotherapy, including EMDR Therapy, and could have happened without LDN. However, as an adjunctive therapy, LDN accelerated psychotherapy progress and played an important role in directly disrupting dissociation, regulating emotions, and stabilizing other PTSD-related symptoms.

Sleep improved as a result of feeling safer at night. It was a relief for her to no longer feel the need to obsessively double-check window and door locks before going to bed. Nightly sleep duration increased from 4 1/2 hours to 5 1/2 or 6 hours, which was ideal for her - her whole life, more than 7 hours typically left her feeling slow and groggy.

As the only female on an otherwise all-male crew, she had been prone to second-guessing her judgment, but she reported that with LDN on board she felt more confident, found it easier to speak her mind assertively, and worried less about what others might think of her and her opinions. When she felt threatened or was highly stressed, if she took 2 mg p.r.n. she was able to keep things in perspective, stay calm, and think clearly.

After taking an LDN dose, ADHD symptoms reduced for about 6 hours, during which time her ability to focus and organize tasks improved: she was able to systematically complete the job at hand instead of multitasking, leaving tasks half done and moving on to the next job. Moreover, she could read books again! Instead of getting distracted after the first paragraph, she was able to stay engaged and enjoy what she was reading.

Somatic Benefits of Adding LDN
Earaches, Hay Fever and Asthma: After years of unsuccessful conventional treatment of chronic earaches due to stenosis (narrow ear canals) and inflammation, the introduction of LDN treatment effectively resolved the issue. The LDN based reduction of hay fever and asthma symptoms significantly improved the status of her earaches, eliminating the need for antibiotic treatments previously required when pollen counts reached high levels. She continued

to take a morning dose of fluticasone along with budesonide and formoterol for asthma, but lacking symptoms, she frequently forgot her evening dose.

Pain From Cysts: Prior to taking LDN, she experienced persistent abdominal pain from an ovarian cyst and pain in her torso and breast from a macro cyst. Soon after starting LDN, pain related to both cysts decreased and eventually diminished to the point that she was virtually pain-free. Two years after starting LDN, the cysts appeared to have stopped growing and she was almost completely pain-free.

Knee Surgery: LDN was her primary pain treatment, providing significant pain relief, while she waited for surgery and during the surgery recovery phase. It reduced inflammation and the use of non-steroidal anti-inflammatory drugs (NSAIDs) as well as opioid pain medications. Before surgery, if she missed her LDN dose, pain increased and she had to increase the use of NSAIDs. She reported, "My surgeon was surprised when he found out that I had only been taking over-the-counter ibuprofen a few times a day even though I was working a 16-hour day with a torn meniscus."

For pain management immediately after surgery, she took a half-dose (2.5 mg) of Hydroco/APAP 5-325 mg (5 mg of hydrocodone combined with 325 mg acetaminophen) before bedtime. She did not take it during the day because she disliked how it made her feel. She resumed LDN therapy the day after knee surgery: 2 mg in the morning, 2 mg in the early afternoon, and 2 mg in the early evening. She discontinued Hydroco/APAP 5-325 four or five days after surgery.

Because naltrexone doses of 50 or 100 mg will interfere with opioid pain medication management, physicians often unnecessarily advise patients to discontinue LDN while taking opioid pain medication. Typical LDN dosing, a mere five or ten percent of a conventional dose, blocks too few opioid receptors to significantly interfere with pain management. In addition, LDN has the potential to prevent building tolerance to opioid pain medication and may prevent constipation associated with opioid pain medications. (Sadee, et al., 2020; Sadee and McKew, 2022; Lang, et al., 2017).

After discontinuing Hydroco/APAP 5-325, she added 200 mg of ibuprofen 3 times a day for approximately a week, after which time she only used ibuprofen infrequently. By the end of the second week, she discontinued all pain medications other than 2 mg of LDN 3 times daily. She set alarms to ensure she did not get too busy and forget her LDN.

She reported that at her two-week post-surgery follow-up, her surgeon was surprised but pleased that she had only taken half doses of Hydroco/APAP 5-325 for four or five days and no longer needed pain medication other than LDN. Six weeks post-surgery, she returned to work with a reduced workload of 12 hours a day. She continued her daily LDN regimen of 2 mg three times daily; if she was extra stressed, she doubled the dose to 4 mg.

Conclusion

This multiple-dose LDN MH protocol contributed to significantly reducing hypervigilance, dissociation, and other PTSD-related symptoms. ADHD-related energy levels, concentration, and focus improved. At the same time, LDN appears to have significantly improved the status of multiple somatic issues and served as an effective pain management tool for acute and persistent (chronic) pain due to earaches, a knee injury, surgery, and pain from cysts.

It should be noted that this case involved acute and chronic pain, both of which benefited from LDN treatment. Her history of long-standing disease states suggests she probably experienced a layering of acute pain and chronic pain. (Grichnik and Ferrante, 1991). That is, traumatic memory of pain likely exaggerated the experience of immediate acute pain. Research shows LDN has the capacity to reduce acute pain, in part due to its anti-inflammatory effects. LDN's capacity to reduce dissociation would have moderated or disrupted the traumatic-memory aspect of chronic pain. (Tesarz, et al., 2019). For a discussion of dissociation and chronic pain see this chapter's introduction.

After the discontinuation of antipsychotics, and the introduction of LDN as an adjunctive to psychotherapy, her somatic and psychological health dramatically improved and she resumed an active, productive life almost completely pain-free.

This case illustrates the importance of closely monitoring patient experience during early adjustment to LDN. Due to this client's extreme sensitivity to medications, she responded best to a dose half of what is often required for effective MH treatment (0.06 mg/kg/b/w); additional fine-tuning was needed to determine when it was most effective to take the medication.

Taking multiple daily doses to gain the full benefit of LDN MH treatment can be a burden, but the advantages usually outweigh the deficits. Its short half-life can also provide an opportunity to manipulate dosing to fine-tune outcomes. Many patients will not require subtle dosing manipulations, but many will benefit from this attention to detail.

Although LDN treatment of somatic issues is associated with a regulation-focused single-dose treatment, this multi-dose suppression strategy added MH gains without compromising regulation-based somatic gains. (See the introduction for a discussion of suppression/disruption vs regulation.)

Patient testimony: "I am no longer in constant pain, I am more focused mentally and able to concentrate on things that matter, and I spend less time hurting and worrying about the past and things that I cannot change. LDN has changed my life for the better and it doesn't have side effects that cause more issues than the supposed benefits of the medication."

PTSD, AS and Comorbid Conditions

Galyn Forster, MS

Abstract
This seven year case study examines the therapeutic benefits of low-dose naltrexone (LDN) in treating a 60-year-old veteran with multiple medical conditions, including post-traumatic stress disorder (PTSD), ankylosing spondylitis (AS), and type 2 diabetes mellitus with associated complications.

The patient, previously dependent on morphine for pain management, was transitioned to LDN therapy while receiving psychotherapy for PTSD. He experienced rapid improvements across multiple domains: reduced pain, improved sleep quality, better emotional regulation, decreased PTSD symptoms, and enhanced management of AS and diabetes-related complications. Improvements were maintained over seven years of continuous LDN treatment.

While distinguishing LDN's specific contributions from concurrent EMDR therapy for PTSD was challenging, the treatment appeared to create synergistic improvements in both psychological and somatic symptoms. This case highlights the potential benefits of LDN as an adjunctive treatment in complex medical cases involving both physical and psychological components.

Introduction
This case study explores the use of LDN as a treatment for post-traumatic stress disorder (PTSD), chronic pain, ankylosing spondylitis (AS, bamboo spine), type 2 diabetes mellitus with neuropathy and erectile dysfunction (ED), and essential hypertension, also known as primary hypertension.

As a trauma-focused psychotherapist, I have found LDN useful as an adjunctive treatment for PTSD and dissociative disorders. Pape and Wöller (2015) published a case series study of 11 patients undergoing treatment for trauma and dissociation in an inpatient setting, which found that the majority experienced a significant benefit from LDN treatment.

As a treatment for PTSD, LDN has a number of advantages: symptom relief from the medication is often immediate, although sometimes it must reach the full dose level of 0.06 mg/kg/b/w to show an effect. It can be an effective pain therapeutic, and it often improves sleep. It has no potential for abuse, side effects are small and transient, and it is non-allergenic and lacks toxicity. In spite of LDN's acknowledged potential as a therapeutic to address multiple medical and psychological issues, it remains grossly under-researched.

Ankylosing spondylitis (AS), also called radiographic axial spondyloarthritis, is a chronic, immune-mediated disease predominantly affecting the axial skeleton, occurring in 0.1% to 0.8% of the population, with onset typically occurring during young adulthood. It is a genetic and environmental based disorder in which cytokine dysregulation characteristically begins with inflammation of the tendons and ligaments connecting to bones. Some individuals experience alternating periods of remission and flare-ups, and in more severe cases fusing of the spine. AS can occur in any part of the spine or the entire spine, often with pain localized to either buttock or the back of the thigh and the sacroiliac joint. There is no cure; treatments focus on slowing the progression of the disease by counteracting long-term inflammatory processes and pain management.

Research has shown LDN to be helpful for treating pain, inflammation and a variety of autoimmune disorders. In recent years it has gained recognition as a promising and safe therapy for pain management, including rheumatic diseases (Younger, et al., 2014; Dara, et al., 2023; de Carvalho and Skare, 2023). Because of this, LDN provided the hope of improving the client's AS and diabetes-related symptoms, as well as better managing pain, which had become unmanageable while opioid pain therapy was being eliminated.

Brown and the pioneering neuroscientist J. Panksepp (2009) observe LDN's "hypothesized disease-modifying effects of enhanced immune functions contradict current medical opinion that immune functions must be globally suppressed to retard the progression of autoimmune diseases. Yet evidence is mounting that LDN may have substantial therapeutic effects in such disorders." Even though it hasn't been researched specifically as a therapeutic for AS, it is an attractive therapeutic to explore as an adjunctive treatment to biologics or, in some cases, as an alternative.

Improving symptoms of erectile dysfunction (ED) has been identified as another potential benefit from LDN therapy, possibly as a result of correcting pathological alterations in central opioid tone (Fabbri, et al., 1989). Independent of the specific mechanism of action, LDN's potential to improve health overall held out hope for improving ED symptoms.

Patient Description

A 60-year-old male veteran with a history of type 2 diabetes mellitus and ankylosing spondylitis (AS), diagnosed with PTSD related to family of origin trauma and battlefield trauma. Symptoms included hypervigilance, anxiety, moderate depression, and irritability. Pain and PTSD tend to mutually magnify one another and this client was no exception. Sleep was disrupted by pain and nightmares, which, in turn, exacerbated PTSD. He rarely got more than five hours of sleep nightly.

Growing up, his basic needs were met, but he was abused and scapegoated by his mother, who seemed to dislike him, was resented by his brother, and rarely saw his father. The fact that he had virtually no memory of his childhood prior to age 12 suggests the abuse at home was extensive.

He was honorably discharged in 1989 after recovering from severe combat-related injuries. Two years later, he was diagnosed with Reiter's syndrome, or what is now called reactive arthritis (ReA). Inflammation and pain in his knees and ankles disabled him for a year before ReA went into remission and he was able to return to nursing and then restaurant management work. Fifteen years later, he was diagnosed with ankylosing spondylitis when a blood test showed that the HLA-B27 gene had turned on. His ribs were becoming fused, making it hard to breathe, and he was in constant pain, with symptoms in his lower back, S-I joint, coccyx, back, neck, and shoulders. He continued to work, managing the pain with high doses of NSAID anti-inflammatories and eventually with 75 mg of morphine 4x daily. When the standard of care changed, and his doctor began titrating his morphine down, pain and mobility got worse. He could no longer listen to clients tell him about their trauma without his own trauma being triggered, and he had to quit working. In 2003, the Veterans Administration (VA) rated him as permanently disabled.

Following are the medical conditions listed in VA documents at the start of treatment with the author: ankylosing spondylitis of multiple sites in spine, primary osteoarthritis (unspecified), joint pain (hand), type 2 diabetes mellitus without complications, male erectile dysfunction, hyperlipidemia, essential hypertension, listeriosis, polyuria and other urinary tract symptoms, dermatophytosis of groin, iridocyclitis NOS, fourth nerve palsy, chronic pain in his neck, second iritis (noninfectious), shortness of breath, esophageal reflux, family HX-GI malignancy, anxiety disorder not otherwise specified, depressive disorder not elsewhere classified.

The biologic etanercept was added to his treatment regimen in 2005, better managing AS symptoms. Eventually, his quality of life improved enough that he was able to return to college, and in 2014, in spite of the handicap of constant pain and opioid pain therapy, he got a graduate degree in mental health counseling. He worked as a clinical rehabilitation counselor until 2017, when morphine was titrated down to a 10th of his original dosage, and the pain became more than he could manage. Shortly after starting therapy with me, he switched from etanercept to secukinumab, a stronger biologic, to better manage his AS. Biologics like secukinumab and etanercept are immunosuppressants that weaken the immune system in order to alleviate symptoms of an underlying autoimmune disorder. While they are helpful for controlling the targeted disease process, they also increase vulnerability to respiratory infections and pathogens.

Further complicating his case, diabetes compromised his health and contributed to neuropathy in legs and feet, as well as erectile dysfunction. When psychotherapy was initiated, his ability to read and think clearly was compromised due to the effects of the opiate pain medications he was still taking.

Diagnosis

He was diagnosed with complex PTSD. His most prominent symptoms included flashbacks of past traumas, repeating traumatic dreams, avoiding reminders of traumatic events, loss of interest in previously-enjoyed activities, irritability, and sleep difficulties. He had a hair-trigger temper, explosive anger, somatic reactions to trauma reminders, feelings of being cut off from others, and difficulty concentrating.

Treatment

Medical care was provided by a Veterans Administration (VA) doctor and a specialist in the community who oversaw treatment of his AS and diabetes. I provided psychotherapy for PTSD and related issues. Previously, he had "talk therapy" from a VA provider.

Psychotherapy focused on managing and resolving symptoms related to battlefield and family of origin trauma. As a corpsman with Navy SEAL training, he was deployed in multiple high-risk combat missions, some of which continued to haunt his dreams and contributed to irritability and a quick temper. He was unable to watch war-related movies without getting emotionally flooded or experiencing flashbacks. In his case, consistent with research and my clinical experience, family of origin neglect and abuse was just as impactful as his combat-related trauma. In the military, to do his job and cope psychologically, he had learned to constructively compartmentalize/dissociate pain and traumatic memories. Most of his combat experiences did not trouble him. What troubled him were memories with an element of moral injury in which innocent civilians were betrayed or killed and a nearly fatal experience in which, as the sole survivor of a failed mission, severely injured, he had to kill or be killed while waiting for rescue.

When he began treatment with me, his VA physician had titrated his morphine sulfate down to 30 mg 3 x daily and soon reduced it to 15 mg 3 x daily, with the goal of completely eliminating opioid treatment. He was worried about how he would deal with increased pain without morphine. His irritability increased considerably and he found himself "barking" at his wife as his pain increased. At the same time, he was hopeful he would regain his former mental quickness and intellect once he was no longer taking an opiate. I encouraged his physician to prescribe a very low dose of naltrexone, 0.5 mg or less, or ultra-LDN, since very small doses of naltrexone can be helpful titrating off of opiates (Mannelli, et al., 2004; Afshari, et al., 2019), but this advice was ignored. After transitioning off of morphine and enduring a badly tolerated trial of gabapentin (his mouth broke out in sores), a trial of LDN was initiated.

LDN Treatment and Outcomes

Pain and Somatic Conditions: He started LDN with a morning dose of 3 mg for three or four days, then increased to 5 mg b.i.d., typically at 10 a.m. and at bedtime. Pain levels quickly decreased, which, in turn, significantly improved the quantity and quality of sleep. He was able to fall asleep faster and, for the first time in 15 years, slept well without having to sit up and move around to deal with the pain. Previously, he had been unable to sleep longer than a total of 5 hours per night, waking up in pain. With LDN, AS-related pain rarely woke him up, and he began sleeping for 7 or more hours, waking rested and ready for the day. He no longer needed to use zolpidem to help with sleep, and cyclobenzaprine HCl, used for muscle spasms, was rarely needed. He continued to take two or three hits of marijuana prior to bedtime.

After three months of LDN treatment, taking 5 mg t.i.d., he was able, for the first time in years, to cross his legs while sitting down. He reported, with delight, that he could again grip a baseball bat and even palm a basketball. After an early history of being an exceptional athlete, regaining these capacities meant a great deal to him.

Coinciding with LDN therapy, he reported having more energy, and the neuropathy in his legs and feet immediately reduced and progressively improved. These gains could be attributed to improved blood sugar levels, with his A1C level dropping by 1.3 points from 10 to 8.7. This may have been directly influenced by LDN, since it has been shown to reduce hyperinsulinemia- induced release of pro-inflammatory cytokines and to reinstate insulin sensitivity, both of which would contribute to improved A1C blood sugar levels (Choubey, et al., 2020; Ang et al., 2014). In addition, naltrexone's apparent ability to disrupt dissociation and addictive behavior may have contributed to more mindful, healthy eating and more conscientious monitoring of blood sugar levels. Better monitoring and maintenance of blood sugar levels and reduced inflammation would also have contributed to improvements in mood and motivation.

A month after starting LDN he began taking walks again. A month later, he reported neuropathy was virtually eliminated in his legs and feet except for a little tingling and numbness in his feet and his toes no longer hurt.

Almost immediately after starting LDN, he announced, 'My sex drive has come back in full force!' He was able to perform better than prior to taking LDN, though not at pre-diabetic levels. Already improving, Type 2 diabetes mellitus symptoms had reduced further, perhaps in part due to LDN's positive impact on inflammation and insulin resistance (Choubey, et al., 2020). While not fully resolved, ED was dramatically improved; he described his ED as two-thirds resolved and no longer an issue. Discontinuing morphine had not significantly altered ED. Improvement in his sleep and overall health likely contributed to better sexual functioning. Initially, his wife 'enthusiastically approved' but after the initial blush, navigating menopause and having grown accustomed to an asexual relationship, his renewed sexual capacity created some relationship tensions, but these were successfully navigated.

Essential hypertension, while not fully resolved, improved after starting LDN, likely due not only to naltrexone's direct biological effects but also to improvement in his ability to regulate emotional reactivity. A growing body of evidence suggests that autoimmunity and inflammation may play a role in the pathogenesis of hypertension (Rodriguez-Iturbe, et al., 2017; Stallkamp, et al., 2023). Hypertension was treated with lisinopril which was discontinued after a few months because it made him cough too much. Since moving to the coast, the reduction of stressors and daily exercise have eliminated the need for pharmaceutical treatment of hypertension.

Psychological Issues: It has been challenging to determine what benefits were the direct result of LDN treatment since, by the time

LDN was introduced, PTSD symptoms were already improving in response to EMDR Therapy. Nevertheless, when LDN was introduced, both he and his wife reported further improvements. Two weeks after starting LDN, not only was he sleeping longer and more soundly, his wife reported he was calmer and less reactive, and he reported his postural orthostatic tachycardia syndrome (POTS) symptoms were improving.

A month after starting LDN, he added a third dose of 3 mg in the afternoon to the 5 mg morning and evening dose. With the additional dose, he was less likely to take things personally or react with anger if his wife 'played the devil's advocate' to something he said when she got home from work. His mood was improved and his wife reported he was laughing more.

At the three-month point, his wife reported he was less easily upset, easier to get along with, and less inclined to ruminate on past family betrayals. He liked that he had a 'longer fuse' before getting angry. She was pleased that he was more likely to manage triggering circumstances without an anger outburst and, when in conflict with her, he was less inclined to abandon the conversation. In the past he would quickly withdraw from a conflict to avoid the possibility of becoming too aggressive and saying something hurtful. EMDR Therapy had helped with this issue, but it is likely that maintaining an adequate serum blood level of naltrexone during waking hours provided additional self-control by disrupting the flight-fight response. He had gotten much better at not over-reacting and was coming to trust himself to manage his emotions far better than in the past.

As an adjunctive to EMDR Therapy, LDN appears to have further helped moderate a pattern of traumatic nightmares. For example, after participating in a veterans trauma survivor group in which he talked about surviving a catastrophic ambush, he had a nightmare of the event, during which he woke up his wife and their dog; but in this case the nightmare didn't keep looping and he went back to sleep. This was progress: it not only didn't loop that night it didn't reoccur in subsequent nights. Having taken LDN before going to bed may have moderated his trauma reaction and probably helped him return to sleep. His recent processing of the ambush experience in therapy (changing remembering from reliving the event in flashback mode to a recollecting of it as over and in the past) likely helped free him up to talk about it in the group. Having LDN in his system that evening would have further increased his ability to feel the reality of his present survival, and increase confidence that he could tell the story without physically re-experiencing it as a flashback. Although he was momentarily distressed, the ease with which he returned to sleep and the fact that the dream didn't keep looping suggest it may have been part of an integrative healing process.

In therapy the following week, reporting about his blood-sugar-spiking love of carbs, he gushed that, 'it was like a light went on!' With LDN on board, he was finding the willpower to say no to carbs. We had done EMDR processing on the issue two or three weeks earlier. Coincidentally, the recent doubling of his LDN dose to 10 mg in the morning and evening, and 6 mg in the afternoon, to better control AS-related inflammation, also appeared to have strengthened his will to eat more healthily. During the same session, he also reported he lost 13 pounds and discontinued his muscle relaxer. Improvements in anxiety, mood and productivity persisted.

Weight loss and treatment of eating disorders appear to benefit from doses higher than conventional LDN levels, possibly because maintaining a full blockade or a constant partial blockade of the opioid system tilts the neurobiological dominance/bias away from habit and addiction towards a fresh awareness of present time experience, towards goals. Complex interactions between the opioid and dopamine systems determine whether habit or reward dominate behavioral choices (Groman, et al., 2019; Mikus, et al., 2022;

Winters, et al., 2017). An adequate blood serum level of naltrexone shifts this balance away from habit (automatic, conditioned responses) towards choices based on current and long-term, value-based rewards, instead of automatically doing what unconscious conditioning (habit or addiction) remembers was rewarded in the past. The biochemistry of habit and addiction may involve, but does not appear to require, trauma-driven dissociative processes.

He reported that periodically, something will trigger a traumatic memory, but the intensity and duration are significantly reduced. This was the case three years after starting LDN, when hearing an automobile backfire triggered a sensory flashback of the iron taste of blood but without feeling extremely startled (probably an implicit memory of smelling blood during a fire fight), but there was no trauma narrative accompanying the sensory experience, and he recovered quickly and went on with his day. We both attributed the progress to his past trauma therapy and LDN's ongoing regulation of real-time emotional reactivity.

Side Effects: The most noticeable side effect he experienced was moderate diarrhea the day he took his first 3 mg LDN dose and the day he increased his dose to 5 mg. In both cases diarrhea resolved within 24 hours. Most clients don't experience diarrhea as a side effect but when they do it typically resolves quickly. He may have been more vulnerable to this side effect because chronic use of opiate pain medications alter opioid system functioning, which could influence gastrointestinal motility. If LDN is discontinued for an extended time period, diarrhea may be experienced briefly when restarting LDN therapy.

Long-Term Use of LDN: He has been taking two or more 5 mg doses of LDN morning and evening for over six years. At the time this study was written, he still had bouts of hypervigilance, but these were short-lived exceptions rather than the rule. He credits EMDR Therapy and LDN for eliminating most of his reactivity and for his

PTSD going into remission. He noted his original family of origin-based trauma has been the most difficult to fully resolve but that this too was better. He no longer had nightmares but could still be triggered by something on television, though it didn't stick with him as it had in the past. He has established a routine of walking for three miles five days a week which has further supported improvements in his mood, AS and diabetic symptoms and has helped keep pain levels and irritability low. In this case, cause and effect are difficult to fully disentangle; there appear to be synergistic interactions between multiple domains, psychological and somatic, wherein an improvement in one domain leads to improvements in other domains.

After he transitioned off morphine, LDN helping him cope with pain and AS symptoms; the benefits were dramatic. At age 65, AS symptoms 'have gotten a little worse,' he is 'very stiff and sore, and still in pain daily.' Nevertheless, secukinumab, reduced stress, increased exercise, and LDN appear to be slowing the progression of AS.

Diabetes is now under control; his A1c is consistently in the low 7s and he takes less insulin than previously. He did a four-day trial of Metformin but discontinued it because he vomited every time he took it.

Sometime after finishing psychotherapy, he was diagnosed with urothelial carcinoma, also known as transitional cell carcinoma (TCC), a type of bladder cancer. It was removed with laser surgery and treated with chemotherapy; he is now free of cancer. While undergoing cancer treatment, he continued his typical twice daily 5 mg LDN dose regimen.

He has taken LDN continuously for seven years, motivated by its therapeutic value in managing AS symptoms and day-to-day hypervigilance and emotional reactivity. In preparing this case study, I asked what he notices if he misses a dose; his response was that he couldn't tell me because he does not miss doses.

Conclusion

This is a complicated case in which LDN appeared to contribute to the disruption of multiple pathological processes, creating a cascade of interdependent improvements in health. Before LDN was introduced, EMDR Therapy was starting to reduce symptoms of PTSD and associated stress. Eliminating opioid pain medication, while initially increasing pain and stress, was essential for paving the way to greater healing. Discontinuing morphine by itself likely supported neurochemical improvements to sleep architecture but before LDN was introduced pain continued to disrupt his sleep. LDN appears to support improved sleep quality in about 50% of patients whether pain is an issue or not. Likely due to LDN moderating pain-inducing inflammation, immediately after starting LDN pain was reduced, and sleep quality and duration dramatically improved.

After he raised his LDN dose to the weight-based target dose of 5 mg (0.06 mg/kg/body weight) and increased the frequency to two or three doses per day, his ability to manage challenging circumstances improved, further reducing his stress load with positive ramifications for both somatic and psychological health. As inflammation and pain levels were reduced and he began feeling healthier, diabetes related symptoms such as blood sugar levels, neuropathy, and ED improved, which in turn led to greater energy, and improved mood and motivation. He began exercising more and eating patterns improved, supporting the positive feedback loops already in motion.

This case provides an example in which alterations to established routines enhanced the treatment of medical conditions. A few months after starting LDN, he had an AS flair which was inadequately treated by his biologic. We found that doubling his target dose from 5 mg to 10 mg b.i.d. or t.i.d. helped moderate AS symptoms, and possibly slowed disease progression. After getting through the inflammation flair, he reinstated his previous dose regimen.

If PTSD had not been a primary focus of LDN treatment, this individual might have been treated with a single daily LDN dose and may have missed out on additional anti-inflammatory benefits tied to multiple daily dosing. But because we were also treating PTSD and emotional volatility, it was necessary for him to take multiple daily doses, due to LDN's short serum blood level half life, in order to disrupt daytime reactivity and other PTSD symptoms. Doubling the size of his dose during AS-related flares appears to have been helpful, and the increased frequency of dosing (b.i.d. or t.i.d.) may have provided additional benefits for management of AS and diabetes-related inflammation; lacking biological testing, we can't say with certainty. Nevertheless, because of how forgiving LDN is as a treatment, and the variability of patient responses to LDN treatment, it makes sense to experiment with different applications. Without increasing dose levels and multiple daily dosing, he might not now be walking Oregon beaches two or three miles daily, five days a week.

As an adjunctive treatment to psychotherapy, LDN helped increase emotional regulation, moderated irritability and anger, reduced over-personalizing and probably helped moderated the intensity and frequency of being triggered into flashbacks. LDN blocks flashbacks of trauma memories as well as trauma-shaped implicit emotional memory by disrupting dissociation (see the chapter introduction). It is difficult to precisely gauge LDN's contribution to the resolution of his trauma since EMDR Therapy clearly played a primary role in moving his PTSD into remission. One would assume that LDN enhanced his ability to self-regulate during the therapy process in a manner similar to how it enhanced emotional regulation and maintaining perspective elsewhere in his life.

Although LDN treatment of somatic issues is typically associated with a regulation-focused single-dose regimen, the multi-dose suppression strategy he used added MH gains and possibly enhanced regulation-based somatic gains. (See the introduction for a discussion of regulation effects vs suppression/disruption effects.)

Endocrine and Hormonal Conditions

Hashimoto's and Chronic Inflammation

Sarah J. Zielsdorf, MD, MS

Abstract

This is a case of a 47-year-old female with Hashimoto's hypothyroidism, persistent weight gain, and chronic body pain, with elevated biomarkers showing chronic inflammation. Treating the hypothyroidism resolved symptoms such as constipation, fatigue, and dry skin but not her chronic inflammation. Low-dose naltrexone (LDN), in addition to other dietary and lifestyle modifications and therapeutic interventions, significantly helped the patient's quality of life via subjective improvements in pain and sleep. LDN has been taken for more than five years with sustained benefit. She has also had significant improvements in her labs, showing a persistent reduction in her chronic inflammatory markers.

Introduction

LDN is used off-label for autoimmune conditions due to its mechanisms of action. Because of its dual ability to increase endogenous beta-endorphin and met-enkephalin levels (also known as opioid-derived growth factor, which has receptors on thyroid cells), LDN is immunomodulatory via its effects on toll-like receptors (TLRs) and T-cells. Hashimoto's Disease is the most common cause of hypothyroidism in the United States and one of the most common autoimmune diseases. A significant percentage of patients do not show improvement or have persistent symptoms even after diagnosis and treatment with thyroid hormone replacement if indicated. This often leads to dissatisfaction with care and poor quality of life. This problem is illustrated with our patient, who presented for fatigue, body pain, and weight gain and was found to have hypothyroidism secondary to Hashimoto's disease, whereby autoantibodies against thyroid tissue can lead to immune-mediated driven destruction of the thyroid gland and permanent hypothyroidism. (McLaughlin P.J. Zagon I.S. 2009).

Patient Description

A 47-year-old female with a past medical history significant for Hashimoto's hypothyroidism presented to our clinic with complaints of fatigue, body pain, and weight gain of approximately 40 pounds (18.14kg). The patient was in her usual state of health until approximately 1 year prior to diagnosis.

History

The patient had a series of significant stressors in 2018, which led to her 2019 autoimmune thyroid diagnosis. She left an abusive marriage of many years, endured financial stress, quit a highly stressful job, moved to a new state in the US, and remarried. She gained 40 pounds, which severely impacted her mental health. In addition, systemic inflammation contributed to the weight loss resistance, as well as the overwhelming extreme fatigue. Prior to her diagnosis, she was physically fit and exercised regularly (biking, running and weight-lifting). In 2019, with no changes to her workout regimen or diet, she gained significant weight, and no amount of calorie restriction, sleep, hydration, or any other treatment helped. In 2021, she had COVID-19, Delta variant, leading to complications of arrhythmia, persistent phantom smells (phantosmia), and persistent hair loss.

Physical Examination Results

Significant physical findings in 2019 included truncal obesity, mild lower extremity edema, noted hair loss/brittle hair, and dry/flaky skin. She reported occasional constipation. Labs as below revealed hypothyroidism, and Hashimoto's by antibody testing as well as findings consistent with thyroiditis on ultrasound.

Test Results

Labs in 2019 were consistent with severe inflammation, including hs-CRP (high sensitive C-Reactive Protein) of 9 mg/L (elevated is greater than 3), and elevated TSH to 11mIU/mL consistent with severe hypothyroidism (normal less than 4.50), laboratory low free T4 at 0.6ng/dL (normal 0.8-1.8) and free T3 1.75pg/mL (normal 2.3-4.2), thyroid peroxidase antibodies greater than 2000 (normal less than 60), anti-thyroglobulin 175 (normal less than 3), elevated lipids including total cholesterol, LDL, HDL, and triglycerides.

Treatment Plan

The patient was treated with synthetic T4 (Levothyroxine) and T3 (Liothyronine), which helped to treat her fatigue but not the chronic pain and inflammation. Given significant persistent symptoms, we initiated LDN therapy in 2019. For autoimmune thyroiditis (Hashimoto's), we start low and slow because thyroid medication may have to be reduced if the thyroid is less inflamed. The patient was prescribed compounded 1 mg scored LDN tablets for cost-effectiveness and ease of use. She started with ½ tablet nightly (0.5 mg) for two weeks. As we assess for side effects (there were none in this case), she increased by 0.5 mg every two weeks until she titrated to max dose 4.5 mg nightly. There was extensive blood work monitoring of thyroid function and other biomarkers at frequent intervals, at first every 6-8 weeks up to quarterly once stable.

Expected Outcome

The expected treatment outcome for improved quality of life with reduced inflammation on Low-dose naltrexone and optimal thyroid hormone/sex hormone management.

Actual Outcome

On optimal therapy with T4 and T3 thyroid hormones, her thyroid labs are stable, she has reduced thyroid antibodies. Hormone replacement therapy has eliminated severe vasomotor symptoms (estradiol patch and oral micronized progesterone). On 4.5 mg of LDN and with supplementation (omega-3 fatty acids, methylated B12/folate, vitamin D3/K2), her hs-CRP (a marker of chronic inflammation) as of 2024 was 1.21 (normal). Lipids were optimal with the achievement of healthy weight loss. With slow titration of LDN dose, the patient states that it took 2-3 months to notice significant improvements in pain levels. One unexpected benefit the patient experienced by taking LDN is better sleep.

Conclusion

This case report illustrates the common and often poorly treated complications of autoimmune disease, which, aside from the systemic effects of the organ(s), tissues, or glands it affects, can drive a chronic inflammatory response. In this case, elevated lipids are a common first symptom of untreated/undertreated hypothyroidism and were historically treated with thyroid medication until proven otherwise.

Autoimmunity-driven inflammation in thyroid disease has no offered treatment or recommendations, leading to further chronic comorbidities. In this case, the treatment of the hypothyroidism does nothing to manage the underlying Hashimoto's disease, and the standard of care is to treat autoimmune vs non-autoimmune-mediated thyroid disease in the same way. LDN should be a standard of care therapy offered to autoimmune patients unless contraindicated or in case of intolerance, given its high safety profile and affordability.

Clinicians should give a trial of LDN 0.5-4.5 mg for up to 18 months as it can take time for maximum efficacy. While LDN alone cannot be ascribed to the nearly complete resolution in inflammatory markers for the patient, and significant diet and lifestyle modifications play an additive and cumulative role, the patient credits LDN for the significant improvements in her overall quality of life.

Autoimmune Progesterone Dermatitis

Marina Straszak-Suri, MD, FRCSC

Abstract

JM is a 34-year-old woman, who has never been pregnant, with a history of severe dysmenorrhea, menorrhagia, and irregular periods since menarche. She underwent various unsuccessful treatments with oral contraceptive pills (OCPs) and Depo-Provera. Subsequently, she developed hives, rashes, oral ulcers, swelling, and joint pain during the luteal phase of her cycle. A diagnosis of autoimmune progesterone dermatitis was established. She then had a cauterization of mild endometriosis, which initially provided some relief. Four years later, she underwent a laparoscopically assisted vaginal hysterectomy, again with initial relief.

Three years later, she was referred for a recurrence of her cyclic pain. She was treated with low-dose naltrexone and immediately experienced a dramatic decrease in both her pelvic pain and cyclic joint pain. Although autoimmune progesterone dermatitis is a rare disorder, we can likely expect its frequency to increase, like all autoimmune diseases. When this condition occurs alongside endometriosis, treating dysmenorrhea becomes very challenging. Low-dose naltrexone should be considered in this context.

Introduction

Autoimmune progesterone dermatitis (APD) is a very rare condition that causes cyclic hives, rashes, and oral ulceration in the luteal phase of the menstrual cycle. In APD, inflammation plays a crucial role as it primarily drives the skin lesions, and joint pain, stemming from an abnormal immune reaction to progesterone. This results in rashes or skin eruptions that often flare up during menstruation when progesterone levels are at their highest. Essentially, the immune system erroneously identifies progesterone as a foreign substance, initiating an inflammatory response in the skin and joints.

Endometriosis is a fairly common condition caused by the displacement of endometrial tissue outside of the uterus, causing dysmenorrhea. Endometriosis is usually treated with progestins, but these are contraindicated in autoimmune progesterone dermatitis.

Patient Description
JM is a 34-year-old G0 who has experienced menorrhagia, severe dysmenorrhea, and irregular periods since her first menstrual cycle.

History
During her menses, JM experienced pain, nausea, vomiting, dizziness, and exhaustion. She was started on the OCP at the age of 16 and was treated for several years, but she continued to have pain and vomiting with her periods. She stopped the OCP after severe vomiting, requiring hospitalization. She took no medications for several years and continued to have pain and vomiting with her periods. She was then started on Depo Provera and then developed circular rashes, oral ulcers, and nasal folliculitis. She discontinued the Depo Provera but continued to have oral ulcers during the luteal phase of her cycle.

After referral to an allergist, she was diagnosed with autoimmune progesterone dermatitis. She also began developing hives, wheezing, skin rashes, swelling, watery stool, swollen lymph nodes, and widespread joint pains during the luteal phase of her cycle. These symptoms were partially treated with bilastine. Her dysmenorrhea was subsequently treated with leuprolide. However, she continued to have dysmenorrhea with vomiting and discontinued due to hot flashes. She went on to have a laparoscopy with cauterization of minimal endometriosis, which initially led to some improvement in her dysmenorrhea.

Four years later, after developing more severe dysmenorrhea, she had a laparoscopically assisted vaginal hysterectomy. Initially, the dysmenorrhea improved after the surgery. She continued to have cyclic episodes of hives, oral ulceration, and skin rashes. She also had several episodes of anaphylaxis in the luteal phase of her cycle with no obvious cause other than progesterone sensitivity. She was prescribed alternating courses of bilastine, montelukast, and rupatadine, which decreased the occurrence of the hives and oral ulcers but did not help with her pain. She was referred to my office with a recurrence of cyclic lower abdominal pain.

Physical Examination
Pelvic examination revealed an absent uterus and diffuse tenderness in both lower quadrants, right greater than left, with no palpable masses.

Investigations
A pelvic ultrasound revealed normal ovaries and a trace of free fluid in the pelvis.

Treatment Plan
Given her autoimmune condition and cyclical abdominal and joint pain, I suggested a trial of low-dose naltrexone. She was prescribed 1.5 mg to take for a week, 3 mg for the following week, and an increase to 4.5 mg daily the following week.

Expected Outcome
The desired outcome was a decrease in the occurrence of both pelvic pain and generalized joint pains, giving the patient a much improved quality of life.

Actual Outcome

According to the patient, the decrease in pain was life-changing. The patient stated that in the previous calendar year, she had missed 67 days of work due to pain. Since starting the LDN, she has only missed 15 days of work due to pain during 11 months of treatment.

Conclusion

Considering the autoimmune nature of APD, LDN was an ideal medication to consider, as it effectively modulates an overactive immune response and reduces the inflammation that causes skin flare-ups and joint pain during menstruation associated with this condition. Given the years this patient has suffered from APD, it is unfortunate that LDN wasn't tried much earlier; it might have prevented the need for invasive procedures and could have spared her extensive suffering.

Chronic Multi-System Symptoms with PCOS

Harpal Bains, MBBS DFSRH PGCAestMed (Dist)

Abstract

This case report emphasizes the complexity of managing chronic, multi-system symptoms exacerbated by hormonal changes, infections, and stress. A 31-year-old woman presented with fatigue, brain fog, joint pain, and digestive issues, which were initially attributed to the discontinuation of hormonal contraception and a viral illness. Subsequent complications, including fibromyalgia-like symptoms and POTS, arose following a second COVID-19 infection. Her menstrual history, which included PCOS and worsening symptoms premenstrually, added an additional layer of complexity to her condition. Combining dietary changes, physical activity, hormonal considerations, and targeted medical therapies resulted in significant improvements. This case underscores the importance of a holistic, patient-centered approach in managing complex, chronic conditions influenced by hormonal cycles.

Introduction

Chronic multi-system conditions, such as fibromyalgia and post-viral syndromes, often present diagnostic and therapeutic challenges, especially when worsened by hormonal fluctuations. Literature suggests that menstrual cycles and hormonal contraception can significantly influence the onset and progression of these conditions. This case details the experience of a 31-year-old woman with a history of PCOS, whose symptoms were intensified by hormonal changes, stress, and viral infections.

Patient Description

A 31-year-old woman has a history of polycystic ovarian syndrome (PCOS) and asthma. She also experienced adolescent acne treated with antibiotics and has used combined oral contraceptives (COC) long-term, which she discontinued due to adverse effects.

History

In November 2020, the patient experienced a sudden onset of fatigue, poor sleep, and brain fog. These symptoms coincided with the discontinuation of the COC, which she had relied on for managing PCOS. The transition was challenging and led to hormonal irregularities and worsened premenstrual symptoms. At the same time, a viral illness (non-COVID) exacerbated her condition.

By 2023, following a second bout of COVID-19, her symptoms included:

- Increased fatigue.
- Fibromyalgia-like symptoms.
- POTS-like symptoms, including dizziness and palpitations.
- Her menstrual symptoms persisted, with a noticeable worsening of fatigue, pain, and mood changes premenstrually.

Physical or Psychiatric Examination Results

- Persistent fatigue, musculoskeletal pain, and TMJ discomfort.
- Stress-related symptoms, including poor quality sleep and complex PTSD.
- No overt physical abnormalities on examination.

Test Results

- Normal laboratory results, including hormonal panels, except for PCOS-related findings (e.g., elevated androgens).
- Stool tests identified mild digestive disturbances linked to gluten and dairy sensitivities.

- Imaging and routine blood tests showed no significant abnormalities.

Treatment Before Coming to Our Clinic:

Medical Interventions:
- Famotidine for brain fog - this improved the brain fog
- Fexofenadine antihistamine when required
- Low-dose antidepressants for anxiety management.

Lifestyle Adjustments:
- Gluten-free and dairy-free diet.
- Pilates twice weekly for musculoskeletal support.

Supplements:
- Vitamin D
- Vitamin B12

Menstrual and Hormonal Support:
- No further support at this time

Mental Health Support:
- Stress management strategies addressing PTSD and work-related challenges.

Current Treatment
- Patient was only interested in a trial of LDN at this point, so no further medical interventions were given.
- Health coaching was provided to guide the patient throughout her journey, especially to navigate any potential side effects of starting LDN.

Expected Outcome
- Reduction in fatigue and brain fog.
- Improved menstrual-related symptoms with a more consistent energy baseline throughout the cycle.
- Enhanced quality of life through better physical and mental health.

Actual Outcome

By mid-2024, on five drops of sublingual LDN (2.5 mg), the patient reported:
- Restorative sleep and improved energy levels.
- Reduced brain fog and enhanced cognitive clarity.
- ADHD symptoms had improved, and they no longer had an intolerance to noise
- Memory improved.
- Skin had improved.
- Significant reduction in joint pain and TMJ discomfort.
- Felt less affected by stress overall
- Improved ability to engage in physical activities such as running and cycling.

However, a flare-up of muscle and joint pain occurred in late 2024, attributed to stress. The patient was managed with low-dose antidepressants by her GP and continued her dietary and exercise regimen. Premenstrual symptoms remained present but were less disruptive. She maintains her current regimen and stays optimistic about gradually increasing her LDN dosage. Despite the recent flare-up, she acknowledges that she is in a significantly better place overall.

Conclusion

This case highlights the interaction between hormonal fluctuations, viral infections, and chronic multi-system symptoms. Managing these conditions requires a multidisciplinary approach integrating hormonal considerations, dietary adjustments, physical activity, and mental health support. For patients with complex hormonal and systemic issues, personalized, holistic care is essential for improving long-term outcomes and enhancing quality of life. Medical professionals should consider prescribing LDN to reduce overall inflammation and modulate immunity, effectively mitigating premenstrual and post-viral symptoms.

Ehlers-Danlos Syndrome

Innovative Management in Ehlers-Danlos Syndrome

Pradeep Chopra, MD, MHCM

Introduction

Ehlers-Danlos syndrome (EDS) is an umbrella term for a group of hereditary soft connective tissue disorders that lead to symptoms such as joint hypermobility, chronic pain, and fatigue. Many individuals with EDS struggle to find effective treatments for pain and inflammation. Recently, low-dose naltrexone (LDN) has emerged as a potential therapy for managing these symptoms. This report presents the case of a patient with EDS who experienced significant improvement in pain and quality of life after starting LDN.

Case Presentation

A 35-year-old woman with a history of hypermobile Ehlers-Danlos syndrome (hEDS) presented with severe chronic pain, muscle fatigue, joint instability, and frequent joint subluxations. The pain in hEDS is typically a mix of nociceptive pain, resulting from joint instability and tissue damage, and neuropathic pain, which stems from nerve involvement and central sensitization. Additional symptoms included skin hyperextensibility, easy bruising, gastrointestinal issues such as bloating and delayed gastric emptying, and autonomic dysfunction characterized by dizziness and tachycardia upon standing (postural orthostatic tachycardia syndrome - POTS).

She also exhibited symptoms consistent with MCAS, including episodic flushing, itching, unexplained rashes, hives, severe allergic reactions, gastrointestinal distress (such as diarrhea, nausea, and cramping), respiratory symptoms like wheezing and shortness of breath, and cardiovascular instability with sudden blood pressure fluctuations. Additionally, she experienced neuropathic pain, which is common in patients with EDS. She also had signs of small fiber neuropathy, including tingling, numbness, and temperature dysregulation. Further complicating her condition, she exhibited features of Chiari malformation, leading to headaches, balance issues, and brain fog, as well as cranio-cervical instability, which contributed to neck pain and neurological symptoms. Lastly, she displayed signs of tethered cord syndrome, resulting in lower back pain, leg weakness, and bladder dysfunction.

Another significant contributor to her chronic pain was Central Sensitization, a condition in which the nervous system becomes hyperreactive, amplifying pain signals and leading to widespread pain, allodynia, and heightened sensitivity to stimuli. This phenomenon is common in EDS patients, making pain management exceptionally challenging. Additionally, low-dose naltrexone (LDN) has been found to reduce mast cell activation, which plays a crucial role in inflammation and allergic responses. (Younger, Jarred, Luke Parkitny, and David McLain. 2014). By stabilizing mast cells and decreasing histamine release, LDN may help alleviate MCAS symptoms, such as chronic pain, fatigue, and hypersensitivity. She had previously tried multiple pain management strategies, including physical therapy, nonsteroidal anti-inflammatory drugs (NSAIDs), and opioids, but experienced limited relief and undesirable side effects.

Treatment with Low-Dose Naltrexone
After researching alternative therapies, the patient's physician recommended a trial of low-dose naltrexone. She started at 1.5 mg per day and gradually increased to 4.5 mg over several weeks.

Results: Within a month of starting LDN, the patient reported notable improvements:

- Reduced Pain: Her widespread musculoskeletal pain decreased, allowing her to reduce her use of NSAIDs.
- Improved Fatigue Levels: She experienced increased energy and fewer episodes of exhaustion. Low-dose naltrexone is believed to enhance energy levels by reducing neuroinflammation and modulating the immune system. By promoting the release of endorphins and reducing overactive glial cell activity in the central nervous system, LDN may help alleviate chronic fatigue associated with EDS. This effect leads to more sustained energy throughout the day, improving overall daily functioning.
- Better Sleep Quality: LDN appeared to help with sleep disturbances, leading to more restful nights. This may be attributed to its role in modulating Toll-like receptors (TLRs) and interleukins, key neuroinflammation regulators. By inhibiting TLR4 and reducing the release of pro-inflammatory cytokines such as IL-6 and IL-1β, LDN may help decrease neuroinflammation and restore normal sleep patterns. This immune-modulating effect contributes to improved sleep quality and overall well-being in patients with EDS. (Brown, Norman, and Jaak Panksepp. 2009).
- Enhanced Mobility: The patient noted improved joint stability, which reduced her risk of frequent subluxations and dislocations. Low-dose naltrexone may also support tissue growth and repair by modulating inflammatory pathways and promoting endorphin release. One key mechanism is its influence on the opioid growth factor (OGF) system, which is crucial in regulating cell proliferation and tissue healing. By modulating OGF and its receptor, LDN may help enhance connective tissue integrity and repair damaged soft tissues, potentially benefiting patients with EDS who suffer from frequent joint instability and soft tissue injuries.

Discussion

Low-dose naltrexone is thought to work by modulating the immune system and reducing neuroinflammation, which may contribute to the chronic pain seen in EDS. While the exact mechanism is still under investigation, LDN has shown promise in other chronic pain conditions, such as fibromyalgia and multiple sclerosis. This case highlights LDN as a well-tolerated and potentially effective treatment for EDS-related symptoms. (Chopra, Pradeep et al., 2017).

Conclusion

For patients with EDS struggling with chronic pain and fatigue, low-dose naltrexone may offer a safe and effective alternative. While further studies are needed to understand its benefits fully, this case suggests that LDN could be a valuable addition to managing EDS symptoms.

Enhancing Quality of Life in hEDS

Rebecca Mass-Krajewski, ARNP-BC, MSN, BSN

Abstract

Low-dose naltrexone profoundly improved the patient's quality of life, allowing her to achieve her goals of active family engagement and an improved ability to handle Activities of Daily Living (ADL) without chronic pain. While setbacks such as menorrhagia and a hip dislocation occurred, they were effectively managed, and the patient resumed her enhanced activity levels.

Introduction

Hypermobile Ehlers-Danlos syndrome (hEDS) is often associated with chronic, hard-to-treat pain that stems from joint instability, connective tissue fragility, and potential central sensitization. Low-dose naltrexone (LDN) can be a transformative therapy for managing pain in hEDS by modulating inflammation and reducing neuroinflammation. Based on the author's extensive experience with complex pain management in hEDS, it is recommended to titrate LDN slowly, increasing by 0.25 to 0.5 mg per week using water titration, especially in patients with neurodivergence, trauma histories, or suspected MTHFR mutations, of which this patient had two confirmed.

Many patients with hEDS also experience mast cell activation issues, which can lead to strong reactions to additives in standard medications. For patients with high suspicion of mast cell activation (e.g., frequent hives, multiple major food intolerances, or strong adverse reactions to pharmaceuticals), starting with compounded LDN can be essential to avoid reactions. This approach was unnecessary for this patient, as she tolerated commercial formulations well during titration. However, she transitioned to compounded LDN upon reaching her final dose to maintain consistency.

The patient describes LDN as life-changing and plans to continue it indefinitely to maintain her improved quality of life. This case demonstrates LDN's efficacy in managing chronic pain and highlights the importance of a comprehensive, individualized approach to complex, multifactorial conditions.

Patient Description

The patient is a 42-year-old married female, a Certified Nurse Midwife, and the mother of a 4-year-old child (G1P1). Her medical history includes Hypermobile Ehlers-Danlos syndrome (hEDS), Bipolar II disorder, PTSD from childhood trauma, polycystic ovarian syndrome (PCOS), ADHD, and Obstructive Sleep Apnea (OSA) effectively managed with CPAP. She experienced significant chronic pain, fatigue, and migraines that limited her ability to engage fully in family and professional life. Her primary goal was to participate in outdoor activities and normal activities of daily living (ADLs) without exacerbating chronic pain.

History

The patient had long-standing issues with:
- Chronic Pain: Persistent pain affecting her shoulders, knees, ankles, and feet bilaterally, worsened by physical activity.
- Fatigue: Significant fatigue, particularly premenstrual, despite effective CPAP therapy and optimal sleep habits.
- Migraines: Frequent and debilitating, often triggered by neck pain and hormonal changes.
- Menstrual Abnormalities: Prolonged menorrhagia secondary to a newly identified fibroid.

- Psychiatric History: Bipolar II disorder and PTSD, well-managed with medications including Wellbutrin, Abilify, and Clonazepam.

Physical or Psychiatric Examination Results
- Physical Exam: Chronic pain was present in multiple joints without acute inflammation or deformity.
- hEDS Criteria: Beighton score of 9/9, positive Steinberg sign, and additional criteria such as stretchy, semi-translucent skin; hyperextensibility; high narrow palate, and piezogenic papules (6 of 12 of Criterion 2 of hEDS evaluation).
- Psychiatric Evaluation: Conducted over 10 years ago and diagnosed Bipolar II disorder and PTSD, stable and managed with ongoing treatment.

Test Results
- Iron Studies: Low-normal iron (55 mcg/dL), TIBC (358 mcg/dL normal), iron saturation (18%), and low ferritin (16 ng/mL).
- Vitamin Levels: Low-normal vitamin B12 (350 pg/mL) and low vitamin D (26 ng/mL).
- Autoimmune and Inflammatory Markers: Normal ANA, rheumatoid factor, anti-CCP, CRP, ESR, Thyroid antibodies, anti-thyroid antibodies (completed in 2019 and 2023)
- Other: normal TSH and Free T4, CBC with differential, Food intolerance test (high intolerance to whey, moderate to casein and cows milk).
- POTS Evaluation: Inconclusive, with occasional tachycardia but no persistent daily symptoms or significant orthostatic hypotension.
- MCAS Investigation: Pending, initiated due to persistent fatigue.

Imaging:
- MRI of Right Shoulder: Evidence of osteoarthritis. Partial tear in the supraspinatus tendon.
- MRI of Right Wrist: Presence of a ganglion cyst. Cartilage loss and an enchondroma.
- MRI of Right Foot: Bunion deformity. Marrow edema with full-thickness cartilage loss. Bipartite sesamoid.
- MRI of Right Ankle: Plantar fasciitis. Paratenonitis of the Achilles tendon. Os navicularis syndrome.
- SIBO Breath Test: Normal results
- Flex Sigmoidoscopy: Noted non-specific inflammation

Treatment Plan
- LDN: The patient started at 0.5 mg and titrated to 4.5 mg using water titration. LDN was trialed independently for the first two months, during which the patient experienced the most significant reduction in baseline pain (40%).
- LDN Update (January 2025): The patient will begin a new dosing schedule of low-dose naltrexone (LDN) at 1 mg in the morning, 1 mg at noon, and 4 mg at bedtime. This adjustment aims to evaluate whether it enhances daytime energy levels while maintaining consistent pain relief throughout the day.

Nutritional Supplements:
- Vitamin D3: 10,000 IU daily for one month, then reduced to 5000 IU ongoing.
- Vitamin B12: Sublingual 2,500 mcg daily.
- Ferrous bisglycinate: Supplementation for low ferritin prior to and worsened during menorrhagia.
- Omega-3 (1 g nightly) and magnesium threonate (480 mg nightly).

Hormonal Management:
- Severe menorrhagia was resolved with Mirena IUD placement, which also reduced migraines significantly.

Lifestyle Modifications:
- Guided meditation added to the morning and bedtime routines reduced stress by 80%. Chiropractic care resolved a hip dislocation that occurred during treatment.

Expected Outcome

The expected outcomes of utilizing LDN included:
- A 5–30% reduction in baseline pain.
- Mild potential improvement in energy levels and mood, possibly related to lower baseline pain.
- Reduced migraines.
- Enhanced ability to participate in outdoor activities and daily life.

Actual Outcome
- Pain Relief: LDN provided a 40% reduction in baseline pain sustained throughout the treatment period.
- Activity Levels: The patient participated in outdoor bike rides with her family 3–4 times per week and walked the dog daily, with no post-activity recovery needed.
- Migraines: Decreased by 30% with LDN alone and were nearly eliminated following amenorrhea achieved with the Mirena IUD.

Setbacks:
- Menorrhagia due to fibroid bleeding was resolved with IUD placement.

- A hip dislocation was successfully treated with chiropractic care.
- Following the resolution of these issues, the patient returned to her new, lower baseline pain.

Conclusion

Low-dose naltrexone (LDN) proved to be a life-changing therapy for this patient with Hypermobile Ehlers-Danlos syndrome (hEDS), significantly improving her quality of life, enabling active family engagement, and demonstrating the importance of a personalized approach to managing complex chronic pain.

Exploring Effective Pain Management in hEDS

Sueanne Baddour, DNP, APRN, FNP

Abstract

Low-dose naltrexone (LDN) can be an effective chronic pain management strategy for patients with hypermobile Ehlers-Danlos syndrome (hEDS). In addition to its efficacy in treating pain, there are many advantages to its use when compared to prescribed opioid pain medication regimens. A case study summarizing the use of LDN for a patient newly diagnosed with hEDS struggling with chronic pain and intermittent opioid medication use is presented. After careful initiation of LDN, the patient successfully discontinued all opioid medication and experienced an improvement in function and overall quality of life.

Introduction

Hypermobile Ehlers-Danlos syndrome is a hereditary connective tissue disorder with joint hypermobility, skin hyperextensibility, and abnormal tissue repair (Malfait et al., 2020). The condition can affect virtually any body system and is often associated with chronic and acute pain, fatigue, gastrointestinal symptoms, orthostatic intolerance, and many other symptoms. Physical therapy and external stabilization, such as bracing and orthotics, are often recommended. Selecting a pharmacologic agent to potentially alleviate several of the condition's symptoms while minimizing adverse effects is ideal.

Low-dose naltrexone (LDN) can be a helpful analgesic option for those with complex, systemic medical conditions, such as fibromyalgia, multiple sclerosis, and inflammatory bowel disease (Kim and Fishman, 2020). LDN's mechanism involves transiently blocking opioid receptors to stimulate endorphin production and modulating glial cell activity to reduce central sensitization, neuroinflammation, and the associated symptoms (Rupp et al., 2023). When compared to traditional, prescribed opioid pain medications, LDN carries much less risk for harm, with a more favorable side effect profile and lack of addictive potential (Driver et al., 2023). LDN may also safely be used concurrently with other prescribed analgesics.

Beyond pain relief, LDN reduces inflammation and modulates the immune system by blocking the production of pro-inflammatory cytokines and upregulating endogenous opioid production, which can provide broader benefits. It may improve sleep, as well as cognitive and fatigue symptoms, and is generally very cost-effective, making it more accessible compared to some opioid medications. The patient presented in this case review was newly diagnosed with hEDS, but suffered from refractory chronic pain that negatively impacted quality of life.

Patient Description
A 61-year-old female Caucasian retired from employment.

History
The patient presented with chronic pain, fatigue, headaches, constipation, shoulder pain, neck pain, jaw pain, bruising, and poor wound healing. There was also brain fog, insomnia, lightheadedness upon standing, dyspnea at times, dry eyes, photophobia, skin sensitivity, stress urinary incontinence, and temperature dysregulation. Physical activity was no longer tolerated, and the patient reported relief from symptoms following attempted physical activity with supine positioning. The reported level of function was rated 5 out of 10.

Established medical diagnoses included fibromyalgia, rheumatoid arthritis, pelvic organ prolapse, perineural cyst, and vitamin D deficiency. Surgical history included bilateral ankle surgeries, right wrist surgery, hysterectomy, treatment of Dupuytren's contracture, cervical laminectomy, placement of spinal cord stimulator with subsequent removal one year later, abdominoplasty, and mammoplasty with revision due to complications during the healing process and incisional hernia.

The primary stated issue was intense achy pain, which had been present daily for decades and worsened later in the day and following physical activity. The pain location was widespread at times but was primarily located in the mandible, trapezius region, cervical spine, and lumbar spine. The patient was followed by pain management specialty and symptoms had not responded well to traditional treatments, nor spinal nerve stimulator trial or cervical laminectomy. Other treatments trialed included multiple epidural steroid injections (ESI), targeted physical therapy after surgical intervention for ankle laxity, and massage therapy.

The patient was taking duloxetine 90 mg daily and oxycodone/acetaminophen 5/325 mg twice daily as needed, without significant pain relief, as well as senna glycoside, doxylamine 25 mg as needed, and a vitamin D supplement. Warm baths provided mild pain relief.

Despite conservative and invasive measures, the patient remained in pain, which significantly impacted their quality of life. Opioid pain medications offered some relief, but also added adverse effects to their lengthy list of symptoms.

Years prior, the patient was given a diagnosis of possible rheumatoid arthritis and offered biologics with methotrexate. These were discontinued shortly after initiation due to adverse effects and lack of clinical benefit. Rheumatology laboratory workup was ultimately non-revealing and imaging of bilateral hands was consistent with degenerative changes.

Physical Examination Results

Relevant examination results included a height of 66" and weight of 120lb. Hypermobility was present in several examined joints with a Beighton score of 8 out of a maximum score of 9. There was mild skin hyperextensibility, dental crowding with narrow palate, arachnodactyly, functional pes planus secondary to ankle laxity, and piezogenic papules to bilateral heels. There were no obvious subluxations and no dislocations.

Test Results

The patient met the clinical diagnostic criteria for hypermobile Ehlers-Danlos syndrome. Laboratory studies included genetic testing for connective tissue disorders and bloodwork. The genetic testing was negative for known pathogenic variants, an expected finding for hEDS. Additional laboratory results ruled out or were negative for anemia, iron deficiency, thyroid disease, autoimmune markers, metabolic imbalance, or inflammatory processes. There was vitamin B12 deficiency and suboptimal vitamin D level. A screening bone density scan was ordered and the report revealed osteoporosis. A baseline echocardiogram was ordered and revealed mild tricuspid regurgitation, mitral regurgitation, mild diastolic dysfunction, normal aortic root, and an estimated ejection fraction of 65%.

Treatment Plan

The patient was educated on pacing techniques to avoid exhaustion and prescribed low-dose naltrexone 0.75 mg orally each evening for 10 days, to increase to 1.5 mg each evening thereafter if tolerated well. They were advised to administer these doses several hours apart from their opioid breakthrough pain medication and were educated on the optimal dosing schedules and time to affect each medication, as these can vary individually. A referral was placed to an orthotics specialty for ankle foot orthoses (AFO) and finger splints, as well as a referral for physical therapy and pelvic floor therapy. Vitamins D, C, B12 complex, and magnesium supplementation were recommended. A bisphosphonate medication was prescribed for the osteoporosis.

Expected Outcome

The expected outcome included attending physical therapy with an hEDS-experienced provider and completing an AFO evaluation. These interventions would provide joint stability and protection. Adding LDN was expected to gradually require adjustments and possibly take months to achieve clinical response.

Actual Outcome

At the five-week follow-up appointment, the patient reported that physical therapy and AFO scheduling were pending. However, there was much improvement in pain, with less heaviness in the shoulders and feeling less fatigued. Pain relief from the LDN was at least comparable to the opioid medication, and the patient had fully weaned off of the opioid altogether. They cancelled the routine follow-up with the pain management specialty and a scheduled ESI procedure. Headaches are now responding to over-the-counter analgesics and there is less constipation. These benefits continued over the next year, and the dose of LDN ultimately stayed at 1.5 mg. After a trial of 3 mg daily offered no additional benefit, the patient was able to enjoy golfing with their spouse once again and felt an overall improved quality of life.

Conclusion

Individuals with hypermobile Ehlers-Danlos syndrome often experience pain from multiple causes and may not tolerate or respond well to certain pain management strategies. Low-dose naltrexone is a safe and effective option for these patients and can be used to transition them away from less safe or less tolerated analgesics. A practical approach is to initiate treatment with 0.5 or 0.75 mg of low-dose naltrexone and gradually increase the dose every 7-10 days as tolerated, up to a maximum of 4.5 mg daily. The optimal dose for an individual is reached when further increases do not yield significant symptom improvement compared to the previous dose, or if adverse effects persist beyond a few days.

Transformative Pain Management in hEDS

Rebecca Mass-Krajewski, ARNP-BC, MSN, BSN

Abstract

Effective pain management for a 46-year-old female with hypermobile Ehlers-Danlos syndrome, autism, and a lifetime of abnormal lab results. In this case study, low-dose naltrexone offers a solution for ineffective mainstream healthcare.

Introduction

Hypermobile Ehlers-Danlos syndrome (hEDS) frequently leads to chronic, challenging pain due to joint instability, fragile connective tissue, and possible central sensitization. Low-dose naltrexone (LDN) can significantly help manage hEDS-related pain by regulating inflammation and minimizing neuroinflammation. Drawing from the author's extensive background in complex pain management for hEDS, it is advised to gradually increase LDN dosage by 0.25 to 0.5 mg each week using water titration. This approach is particularly crucial for patients with neurodivergence, histories of trauma, or suspected MTHFR mutations, as seen in this patient who had two confirmed mutations.

Many individuals with hEDS often face mast cell activation problems, resulting in heightened sensitivity to additives in typical medications. For those who show significant signs of mast cell activation (such as recurrent hives, several major food intolerances, or severe negative responses to drugs), initiating treatment with compounded LDN may be crucial to prevent reactions. This patient did not require this approach; she handled commercial formulations well during titration. However, she switched to compounded LDN upon achieving her final dosage for consistency.

The patient considers LDN transformative and intends to use it long-term to sustain her enhanced quality of life. This case underscores LDN's effectiveness in addressing chronic pain and emphasizes the necessity of a thorough, personalized strategy for complex, multifaceted conditions.

Patient Description

The patient is a 46-year-old married female, a stay-at-home wife and mother who homeschools her younger child. Diagnosed with autism at age 42, she has two children (G2P2) with ADHD and autism. She presented to the clinic to explore whether hypermobile Ehlers-Danlos syndrome (hEDS) could explain her lifetime history of joint dislocations and chronic pain. She'd read of the hEDS connection to autism online.

The patient has a long-standing history of poor experiences with mainstream medical care. Numerous providers attributed all her health complaints to her weight, offering limited options such as nutritionist referrals or bariatric surgery. This approach led to a significant avoidance of medical care, with the exception of psychiatric treatment. The COVID-19 pandemic facilitated her access to care via telemedicine, enabling her to seek help without facing in-person stigmatization.

History

She was a chronically sick child who took a great deal of antibiotics, and was later diagnosed with asthma. She began to have joint dislocations and pain in elementary school.

The patient reported the following key symptoms and history, which have worsened since she was in elementary school:

- Hands and Fingers: Symmetrical pain in finger joints, particularly the middle knuckles, worsened during summer with swelling. The pain extended into the palms, severely limiting fine motor tasks like crocheting and impacting daily living and leisure activities.

- Chronic Pain and Joint Instability: Severe chronic pain and frequent dislocations affecting the hands, shoulders, hips, knees, and ankles.
- Mental Clarity and Fatigue: She has a persistent lack of mental clarity, which bothers her significantly more than her mild fatigue. Despite feeling she sleeps well for sufficient hours, she struggles with cognitive fog. Her spouse has not observed snoring or any notable disturbances in her sleep.
- Shoulders: Recurrent partial dislocations, predominantly on the right side, triggered by activities like rolling over in bed or walking the dog. The left shoulder dislocated less frequently. Pain occurred during and after dislocations.
- Hips: Frequent dislocations, especially the right hip during specific activities like sex, causing sharp pain and residual soreness.
- Knees: Persistent pain with occasional buckling and a history of sprains lasting weeks.
- Ankles: Frequent rolling of ankles with prior ligament tears and ongoing instability.

Physical Examination Results
- Chronic Pain: Present in multiple joints without signs of acute inflammation or deformity.
- Morbid Obesity: BMI 50+

hEDS Criteria:
- Beighton Score: 5/9.

Additional Criterion 2 Features:
- Stretchy, semi-translucent skin.

- Skin hyperextensibility.
- High, narrow palate.

Bilateral piezogenic heel papules (>5):
- Meets 5+ of 12 features in Criterion 2 of hEDS evaluation.
- No signs of other connective tissue disorders were identified during the evaluation, and genetic testing was deemed unnecessary.
- White Blood Cell Count: Persistently elevated for 10 years, leading to multiple investigations that did not provide definitive answers.
- Nutritional Absorption: Multiple providers indicated concerns regarding poor absorption of vitamins and nutrients, which could contribute to chronic symptoms.
- Autism: Diagnosed with autism at age 42 with neuropsychiatric evaluation.
- Moderate Recurrent Depression: Diagnosed with depression in her 20s, which worsened in 2019 and is now stable.

Test Results and Other Investigations
Sleep Study: A new sleep study conducted by a specialty dentist in 2024 ruled out obstructive sleep apnea (OSA) but identified jaw misalignment as a potential factor impacting sleep quality.

Dental Device: A custom dental device was prescribed to address the jaw misalignment. Initially, the device caused significant jaw discomfort, disrupting sleep for over a month. After adjustments, the patient noted slight improvements in energy levels the following day, suggesting a marginal benefit from its use.

Barriers to Care: Progress and investigations have been substantially hindered by:
- Long referral times.

- Providers lacking expertise in hypermobile Ehlers-Danlos syndrome or histamine-related issues.
- Front office miscommunication or lack of communication.
- Lab redraws in May 2024 misprocessed ESR and CRP, so it is unclear how fast LDN helped normalize labs.

Test Name	Aug-23	Dec-23	Apr-24	May-24	Oct-24	Dec-24
ANA	Positive 1:40				Normal	
C-Reactive Protein	31	31.4			18.7	
Sed Rate by modified Westergren	46	50		Sample Issue, DNR		
White Blood Cell Count	12.9	9.7			8.5	
Tryptase			5.1			
Histamine			5.2		1.6	
Prostaglandin D2				44		
Iron (40-190 mcg/mL)	37	42			36	36
Ferritin (16-232 ng/mL)	40	29			31	31
TIBC (250-450 mcg/dL)	295	326			308	308
Iron Saturation (16-45%)	13	13			12	12
Vit D (30-100 ng/mL)	43				45	

The patient experienced elevated Immunoglobulin G subclass levels on three occasions, with values ranging between 214 and 250 mg/dL (normal range: 4–86 mg/dL). Despite this consistent abnormality, the specialist expressed no concern about these findings when she saw an immunologist/allergist after a 6-month wait. However, during the visit, the discussion primarily revolved around ruling out mast cell activation syndrome (MCAS), which was not the primary reason for her referral or appointment. Still, the patient could not redirect the provider.

Additionally, a Vitamin B panel revealed that all lab results were at the low end of the normal range, further supporting previous investigations indicating that the patient does not absorb vitamins or nutrition effectively. This pattern may contribute to her broader health challenges and warrants consideration in her overall care plan.

Treatment Plan
The treatment plan focused on managing the patient's chronic pain, histamine/mast cell issues, and sensitivity to medications. Key components included:

- Low-Dose Naltrexone (LDN): Initiated at a very low dose of 0.25 mg (October 2023) and slowly titrated to the maximum tolerated dose over 3 months to address chronic pain while minimizing potential adverse reactions.
- hEDS: The patient is not ready to consider physical therapy.

Histamine/Mast Cell/Inflammation Management:
- Famotidine 40 mg daily

Consolidated recommendations from prior allergist and psychiatric evaluations into:
- Symptom management with targeted antihistamines and mast cell stabilizers.
- Nutritional support with supplements such as omega-3, vitamin D, and zinc reduces inflammatory triggers and supports systemic health.

Medications:
- Sertraline: 50 mg once daily for mood
- Rexulti: 0.5 mg once daily for mood
- Montelukast: 10 mg once daily for asthma
- Metformin: 500 mg once daily for weight management related to other medications (no diabetes)
- LDN

Supplements:
- Omega-3: 3000 mg once daily for eye health and pain
- Vitamin B Complex:
- Vitamin E: 268 mg once daily for eye health
- Vitamin D: 5000 IU
- Zinc: 50 mg once daily for eye health
- Lutein: 20 mg once daily for eye health
- Potassium/Magnesium: Potassium (99 mg) and Magnesium (180 mg) once daily for eye health and pain
- Collagen: 2.5 g once daily for nail health

Expected Outcome

On LDN, the patient was expected to experience a 5–30% reduction in baseline chronic pain. We will see a reduction in the continually elevated WBC, ESR, and CRP.

Actual Outcome

She tapered up 1 to 1.5 mg per month. She felt no improvement from 4-4.5 mg but did have new mild nausea. Dropping back down to 4 mg she did not, and she has maintained that dose for a year.

Within three months, the patient reported, "I no longer have hand or finger pain. I can crochet every day. I do not think about my hands anymore." This outcome far exceeded expectations, with complete resolution of hand and finger pain, allowing her to resume meaningful activities. She can now walk her dog daily due to the elimination of hand/finger pain, and reduced knee and hip pain.

She still has dislocations, but they bother her less overall due to reduced pain levels.

WBC normalized for the first time in 10 years within 12 months of starting LDN and supplements. ESR and CRP both reduced chronic elevation by 50%.

Conclusion

Low-dose naltrexone proved to be a transformative treatment, eliminating chronic debilitating hand and finger pain that had previously restricted the patient's ability to perform ADLs and enjoy leisure activities. This case underscores the importance of considering therapies like LDN for managing complex chronic pain, especially in patients with a history of medical avoidance and stigmatization, due to minimal side effects with a broad range of potential benefits. LDN has been instrumental in enabling daily life with minimal pain for a patient with Hypermobile Ehlers-Danlos while reducing inflammation, as evidenced by blood work trends.

Telemedicine was pivotal in enabling this patient to access care, highlighting its value for individuals with barriers to traditional healthcare settings.

Acknowledgements

We would like to express our sincere gratitude to all the authors who contributed their case studies—this book would not have been possible without their invaluable help and support.

Special thanks also go to Paula Johnson for her meticulous editing and typesetting.

And last, but not least, thank you to you, dear reader, for taking the time to engage with this book. We hope you find the information within of great value to you.

Author Biographies

Paul S Anderson, NMD

Dr Anderson is a recognized educator and clinician in integrative and naturopathic medicine with a focus on complex chronic illness, and cancer. In addition to three decades clinical experience, he also was head of the interventional arm of a US-NIH funded human research trial using IV and integrative therapies in cancer patients. He founded Advanced Medical Therapies in Seattle, Washington, a clinic focusing on cancer and chronic diseases and now focuses his time in collaboration with clinics and hospitals in the US and other countries.

Former positions include multiple medical school posts, Professor of Pharmacology and Clinical Medicine at Bastyr University and Chief of IV Services for Bastyr Oncology Research Center.

He is co-author of the Hay House book "Outside the Box Cancer Therapies" with Dr Mark Stengler, and the Lioncrest Publishing book "Cancer… The Journey from Diagnosis to Empowerment.". He is also co-author with Dr's Osborne and Carter of the IV textbook "A Scientific Reference for Intravenous Nutrient Therapy".

Sueanne Baddour, DNP, APRN, FNP

Dr Baddour is a family nurse practitioner of more than eleven years. She has a background in primary care and academia. She founded a private hypermobility practice that reaches patients across several states. Her clinical focus and passion are for underrecognized, underserved, and complex patient populations.

She actively participates in The Ehlers-Danlos Society's EDS ECHO clinician program. She dedicates her time to serving those living with hereditary connective tissue disorders, such as hypermobile Ehlers-Danlos syndrome (hEDS), and associated conditions, such as dysautonomia and mast cell activation syndrome.

Harpal Bains, MBBS, DFSRH, PGCAestMed (Dist)

Dr Bains has been immersed in the world of bioidentical hormones, functional medicine and environmental medicine for the past 10 years after following a conventional path within the NHS completing her basic surgical rotation. She is now focussed on longevity medicine with an emphasis on prevention and screening for both well and ill patients.

Dr Bains is an advanced BHRT practitioner and has been trained under Dr Neal Rouzier. She is trained in Psychosexual Medicine and has completed her Diploma in Sexual and Reproductive Healthcare. She is also an advanced practitioner in Aesthetic Medicine. She found that her core skill set was in unravelling complex medical puzzles and putting together protocols that could be adapted to individuals based on their unique history, mindset and personality.

Currently, besides longevity medicine, she also focuses on patient psychology, brain retraining and the concept of 'helping the body help itself'. She trains other medical practitioners in her methodology and protocols within her practice. This has helped give her the time to focus on discovering and exploring new ideas and where relevant, incorporate them within her practice.

She fervently believes that as medical practitioners, we have to constantly be curious, ask questions and have intellectual humility. Her goals for the future include more speaking and mentoring opportunities, training and writing.

Jeff Barris, PharmD

Dr Barris is a Doctor of Pharmacy and owner of Pacifica Pharmacy, earned his Doctorate of Pharmacy degree in 1970 from USC as one of only 150 graduates and the very first class to obtain the class of doctorate in pharmacy.

At 16, he developed a passion for compounding while learning the ropes at a small compounding pharmacy in West Los Angeles, working with individuals and customizing formulas. He eventually opened a compounding pharmacy in 1983 in Torrance, California. He connected with PCCA, an organization specializing in compounds, a partnership where collaboration and knowledge were key.

Jeff remains on the cutting edge of medicine, health, and wellness, focusing on integrative health and prioritizing patient education. He is certified in hormone replacement therapy (HRT) and is an expert in low-dose naltrexone (LDN) and nutrition. Today, Jeff is consulting with patients, suggesting options and solutions for their healthcare needs.

Matthew Bennett, MD

Dr Bennett is an orthopedic spine surgeon and functional medicine expert who has dedicated his career to helping individuals overcome chronic pain and unlock their full potential. With a foundation in Nutritional Sciences from Cornell, fellowship training at the multidisciplinary Texas Back Institute, and board certifications in orthopedic surgery and regenerative medicine, Dr Bennett brings a unique, integrative approach to healing. His work bridges the best of medicine, movement, and mindset, empowering patients to reclaim their lives and thrive beyond pain through resilience and transformation.

Edyta Biernat-Kałuża, MD, PhD

Dr Biernat-Kałuża is a consultant rheumatologist, internal medicine doctor. PhD title: "The Meaning of Seronegative Arthritis in Orthopaedic Practice." She places an emphasis on the individualization of treatment, applying various therapeutic methods within academic medicine, as well as lifestyle medicine, personalized nutrition, orthomolecular and mitochondrial medicine, naturopathy, and LDN treatment.

Member of the Scientific Councils of the Foundations: "We Know What We Eat" and "Multis Multum"; a member of ACR - American College of Rheumatology and PTR - Polish Rheumatology Society; the sole Polish representative in G-CAN - Gout, Hyperuricemia, and Crystal-Associated Disease Network; multiple participant at the Cleveland Clinic conferences on Preventive Medicine; a member of Advisory Board in start-up Smarter Diagnostics, which introduces AI software for image diagnostics in orthopaedic/sport medicine and realises European Space Agency grant and cooperates with NASA. Author/coauthor of numerous presentations and articles in Polish and international literature. Lecturer at LDN conferences about LDN in rheumatology.

Pradeep Chopra, MD, MHCM
Dr Chopra is currently the Director of the Center for Complex Conditions and an Assistant Professor at Brown Medical School. He completed his training in Anesthesia and Critical Care, along with a Fellowship in Pain Medicine at Harvard Medical School. He has a particular interest in chronic complex pain conditions and their associated co-existing conditions. His contributions to the field include several publications, and he serves on the editorial board of a journal focused on pain management. Additionally, he is a member of the medical advisory board for several chronic pain conditions and is the former chairman of the EDS International Pain Consortium. He has received numerous national awards, including the Compassionate Care Award, Lifetime Achievement Awards, and the Humanitarian Award.

Sebastian Denison, RPh

Sebastian worked at Northmount Pharmacy in North Vancouver for 11 years, specializing in HRT, veterinary, pain and sports compounding. He was also the manager of Pharmacy Operations for the 2010 Vancouver Winter Olympic/Paralympic Games and then the manager of the Whistler Olympic Village Polyclinic Pharmacy.

In addition to his role as a PCCA clinical compounding pharmacist, Sebastian works with both the U.S. and Canadian CORE compounding training education teams and the pharmacy student education team.

Sebastian also speaks at physician, pharmacist and other healthcare professional education symposiums and events. He has recently lectured for the American Academy of Anti-Aging Medicine on Nutrition and Pain, Pharmacy Compounding and Collaborative Practice, and Alternative Uses for Naltrexone.

Galyn Forster, MS, PLC

Galyn is a Licensed Professional Counselor practicing in Eugene, Oregon since 1988. He earned an MS in Counseling Psychology from the University of Oregon. He works with adults, youth, and couples, focusing on a wide range of issues, including complex trauma, dissociation, anxiety, attachment issues, physical pain, and traumatic brain injury. His theoretical orientation for clinical practice is eclectic, with an eye to integrating recent neurobiological findings into his treatment.

Central to his practice are Eye Movement Desensitization Reprocessing Therapy (EMDR), Coherence Therapy, Acceptance and Commitment Therapy (ACT), Sensorimotor Therapy, and LENS neurofeedback. He began working with patients prescribed low-dose naltrexone (LDN) as an adjunctive treatment to psychotherapy in 2010. Since then, he has helped over 100 clients in their exploration of LDN as an adjunctive treatment for mental health issues. He has presented locally and internationally on the topic of using LDN as an adjunct to psychotherapy.

Todd Hill, ABPN

Dr Hill, a psychiatrist for over 22 years and board-certified in General Psychiatry by the Academy of Psychiatry and Neurology, practices psychiatry and TMS at NeuroWellness Spa and serves as their medical director in Westlake and Encino locations.

Before his time at NeuroWellness Spa, he owned his private practice for 10 years, was on staff as a consultation psychiatrist for multiple Kansas City hospitals, and served as the Medical Director of Psychiatric Services at one of the largest hospitals in the Kansas City Metro area. As a psychiatrist who believes in education, he served as Assistant Professor and Department Chair of Psychiatry at his alma mater, Kansas City University of Medicine and Biosciences. Dr Hill has been working with low-dose naltrexone and helping patients with mood disorders for over 5 years now and continues to help patients live their best lives.

Arash Jalali-Sohi, Medical Student

Arash is originally from the San Francisco Bay Area in Northern California. He completed his Bachelor of Science degree in Neurobiology, Physiology, and Behavior at the University of California, Davis.

He has previously conducted basic science research in the fields of plant pathology and COVID-19 assay development. Arash has also worked in clinical research in neurology, pulmonology, and urology. He is currently a medical student at Weill Cornell Medical College

Meredith Kushner, MD, MS

Dr Kushner is a dedicated anesthesiology resident at NewYork-Presbyterian Hospital/Weill Cornell Medicine in New York City. She earned both her Doctor of Medicine (MD) and Master of Science (MS) degrees. Prior to her residency, Dr. Kushner was an active medical student at Loyola University Health System in Chicago. In her current role, she is affiliated with esteemed institutions such as Memorial Sloan Kettering Cancer Center and the Hospital for Special Surgery. Dr. Kushner has co-authored several publications in the field of anesthesiology, contributing to advancements in medical knowledge. Her professional interests encompass perioperative patient care, pain management, and medical education

Rebecca Mass-Krajewski, ARNP-BC, MSN, BSN

Rebecca is an Advanced Registered Nurse Practitioner and Medical Detective at The EDS Clinic PLLC. She specializes in Hypermobile Ehlers-Danlos syndrome (hEDS), Postural orthostatic tachycardia (POTS), Mast Cell Activation Syndrome (MCAS), and related disorders. She became the person she needed because there was no one to guide her on her own health odyssey.

Drawing from her total body framework, Rebecca guides patients with complex chronic illnesses toward healing and renewed confidence. She understands the deep frustration of those struggling with multiple symptoms, medical uncertainty, and decision overwhelm. By carefully mapping each patient's health journey from the beginning, she uncovers hidden connections and contributing factors that others may have missed. This insight allows her to develop individualized treatment strategies that blend conventional medicine, supplementation, and mind-body practices. Through this comprehensive approach, her patients consistently report significant improvements in pain levels, energy, and overall wellbeing.

Neel D. Mehta, MD

Dr Mehta, MD, is the Division Chief of the Weill Cornell Pain Management Center and an Associate Professor of Clinical Anesthesiology at Weill Cornell Medical College. He also serves as a Co-Director of Och Spine at Weill Cornell Medicine. He is the Immediate-Past President of the Eastern Pain Association and Secretary of the New York Society of Interventional Pain Physicians.

Dr Mehta completed his fellowship in Interventional Pain Medicine in the Tri-Institutional Pain Medicine Fellowship at NewYork-Presbyterian Hospital/Weill Cornell Medical Center, Hospital for Special Surgery, and Memorial-Sloan Kettering Cancer Center.

Scott Mortenson, MD, PA, MPAS, MALT, EMT-P

Dr Mortensen is a physician, researcher, and philanthropist specializing in regenerative medicine, peptide therapies, and neuroimmune modulation. With over 25,000 hours of direct patient care, he serves as Clinical Director at Holtorf Medical Group and CPC USA, where he develops cutting-edge protocols for chronic inflammation, neuroprotection and longevity.

His medical career spans mission-critical roles in search and rescue, disaster relief, and extreme environments, including serving as a medic on an Everest summit team and leading operations in Haiti, Alaska, and Africa. As Chief Medical Officer on an unprecedented Arctic Row Ocean expedition, he secured a Guinness World Record.

Dr Mortensen is currently at the forefront of low-dose naltrexone (LDN) research, collaborating with Dr Kent Holtorf to refine LDN protocols for autoimmunity, chronic pain, and mental health. His work explores AI-driven personalized medicine and the intersection of immune modulation and neuroinflammation to unlock new treatment paradigms.

A dynamic speaker, author, and educator, Dr Mortensen is passionate about empowering patients to reclaim their health through tailored therapies, resilience, and informed decision-making. His expertise, combined with a relentless pursuit of innovation, positions him as a leading voice in the future of LDN and regenerative medicine.

Greta Niemela, MD

Dr Niemela earned her medical degree from the University of Washington School of Medicine in 2023. After successfully completing her studies, she began her residency in Anesthesiology at Weill Cornell Medical Center, where she is currently engaged in advanced training. Dr. Niemela is committed to developing her skills in this critical field and is dedicated to providing high-quality patient care throughout her residency.

Rachel Noonan, PharmD

Dr Noonan received her Bachelor's in Biochemistry from the University of Maine in 2007, and earned her Doctor of Pharmacy from Massachusetts College of Pharmacy and Health Sciences in 2010. As a pharmacist and patient care advocate with over 15 years of professional experience, she has thrived in both commercial and compounding practice.

Since joining Belmar Pharma Solutions in 2021, Rachel dedicates her work to championing women's hormonal health and wellness and educating patients and providers about the benefits of customized compounds. As Belmar's Clinical Research and Content Marketing Pharmacist, Rachel creates data-driven webinars, investigates and composes clinical content, and leads expert consultations. Rachel believes in great food and even better fiction.

Rehana Sajjad, MD, FACOG, ABAARM

Dr Sajjad graduated from medical school in 1971 and began her career in Pakistan, where she worked for 4-5 years, including house jobs until 1976. Her journey then took her to Iran, where she served in the Ministry of Health for four years until 1980, navigating through the challenges of the Iranian Revolution during her tenure. In 1981, Rehana relocated to Dubai, continuing her work with the Ministry of Health until 1992. During this time, she successfully passed the MRCOG Part 1 exam.

In pursuit of further growth, Rehana moved to the United States, where she completed her residency in Obstetrics and Gynecology. From 1992 to 2000, she was affiliated with Queens Long Island Medical Group. Following this, she established her private practice, which she continues to manage today. In 2018, she enhanced her expertise by becoming board-certified in Integrative and Functional Medicine. Fluent in Punjabi, Urdu, Hindi, Persian, and English, Rehana Sajjad combines her diverse cultural background with extensive medical experience to provide comprehensive care to her patients.

Yusuf (JP) Saleeby, MD, CTP

Dr Saleeby is an Integrative and Functional Medical Physician. He is an author of books and chapters in books on Functional and Holistic Medicine. Dr Saleeby is the Medical Director of two centers in South Carolina (Carolina Holistic Medicine) and founder of the Priority Health Academy (PHA) a non-profit educational arm of the practice. His Academy provides education and training in functional medicine/healing and assists those wishing to establish centers similar in the USA and Canada. He is a clinical professor in functional medicine and biomedical ethics for the PHA. He is an avid warrior for medical freedoms and patient advocacy. Senior Fellow with the FLCCC (now the IMA) and advisor and co-chair of the educational committee for the BODY Healthcare. Advisor to the LDN Research Trust.

He retired from Emergency Medicine after 17 years to focus on a more holistic approach to patient care. He has an interest in Medical History and lectures on the American Civil War topics. Dr Saleeby is a member of medical organizations such as: IFM, ILADS, AARM, ISEAI and in association, and Senior Fellow to the IMA (FLCCC) and advisor to the BODY Healthcare, the LDN Research Trust. He founded the Priority Health Academy in 2018 teaching others a form of functional medicine.

Marina Straszak-Suri, MD, FRCSC
Dr Straszak-Suri is an experienced OBGYN and a dedicated educator with over 30 years of clinical and teaching experience as an Assistant Professor at the University of Ottawa Faculty of Medicine. She combines her medical expertise with a passion for evidence-based, holistic approaches, naturally empowering individuals to optimize their reproductive health. Dr Marina enjoys teaching and mentoring the next generation of medical professionals while staying at the forefront of scientific innovation. She emphasizes the importance of lifestyle improvement to achieve health and longevity and has been an LDN prescriber for years. Dr Marina is currently writing a book on optimizing fertility naturally, in which she discusses the use of LDN in this context. Inspired by her journey as a mother, she shares cutting-edge insights and practical strategies to help readers navigate the complexities of conception and pregnancy. Through her compassionate and educational approach, she aims to demystify fertility and provide the tools to build healthier, thriving families.

Sahar Swidan, PharmD, ABAAHP, FAARFM, FACA
Dr Swidan is President and CEO of NeuroPharm and Former CEO of Pharmacy Solutions in Ann Arbor, MI and Adjunct Associate

Professor of Clinical Research and Leadership at George Washington University School of Medicine and Health Sciences, and Adjunct Clinical Associate Professor of Pharmacy at Wayne State University.

She received her Doctor of Pharmacy degree and completed a 3-year research Fellowship in Bio-Pharmaceutics and Gastroenterology at the University of Michigan. Following her fellowship, she was Director of Pharmacy at Chelsea Community Hospital and the clinical pharmacist for the inpatient head and chronic pain service.

Dr Swidan is board certified and an advanced fellow in anti-aging and regenerative medicine. She is an internationally renowned speaker in the areas of pain management, headaches, and HRT. She has authored several book chapters, articles, and patient education material in head and general pain management and personalized medicine.

Most recently, Dr Swidan has contributed in authoring "Metabolic Therapies in Orthopedics, Second Edition". This edition provides continued knowledge on how optimizing metabolic pathways can improve the success of regenerative therapies through emerging technologies, integrative approaches, clinical research, and compelling evidence from over 30 experts. Dr Swidan provides key insight in the areas of drug-related muscular pain and sarcopenia and the effects of hormones on the musculoskeletal system.

Dr Swidan Co-Edited and Authored a book with many thought leaders from around the globe titled Advanced Therapeutics in Pain Medicine which aids clinicians in advancing their current toolbox in the treatment of various pain syndromes.

Leonard Weinstock, MD, FACG
Dr Weinstock was born and raised in New York and moved to St. Louis in 1985. He received his medical training in Rochester, New York and completed his Gastroenterology fellowship at Washington

University. He is Board Certified in both Internal Medicine and Gastroenterology.

He is an Associate Professor of Clinical Medicine and Surgery at the Washington University School of Medicine. Dr Weinstock's lectures and research have been presented at national and international conferences on small intestinal bacterial overgrowth, restless legs syndrome, rosacea, and mast cell activation syndrome.

Dr Weinstock provides individualized care to all adult patients with gastrointestinal disorders. His clinical practice emphasizes colon cancer screening, therapeutic video endoscopy, motility disorders, diagnosis and management for irritable bowel syndrome, and comprehensive management of inflammatory bowel disease.

Dr Weinstock is married and has twin daughters. In his spare time, he enjoys cooking, drawing, and being a grandfather to 3 boys.

Sarah J. Zielsdorf, MD, MS, ABIM, IFMCP

Dr Zielsdorf is a certified practitioner in Functional Medicine and is board-certified in internal medicine. She is the Owner and Medical Director of Motivated Medicine, an innovative consultative medical practice located in West Chicago, Illinois. She is a skilled diagnostician, microbiologist, and passionate educator. Dr Z specializes in chronic illnesses, particularly autoimmune diseases, and is deeply committed to women's health, with a focus on hormone management—including thyroid, sex hormones, adrenal health, and more.

Additionally, Dr Zielsdorf serves as a medical and research advisor and the education director for the LDN Research Trust. She teaches internationally and created the 2020-2024 LDN Guides. Dr Z is also an author featured in Volumes 2 and 3 of the LDN Book and New Horizons. The Motivated Medicine approach she developed (and continues to refine) is based on Translational Medicine, which connects current clinical research from around the world with the direct care provided by physicians. Dr Zielsdorf's open-minded approach to treatment is informed by data, advanced diagnostic testing, whole-body wellness, conventional medicine, and much more.

References

– Abhinav Choubey, Khyati Girdhar, Aditya K Kar, et al., 2020. "Low-Dose Naltrexone Rescues Inflammation and Insulin Resistance Associated with Hyperinsulinemia." *Journal of Biological Chemistry* 295 (48): 16359–69. https://www.jbc.org/article/S0021-9258(17)50455-X/fulltext.

– Afshari, Reza, Majid Khadem-Rezaiyan, Hoda Khatibi et al., 2019. "Very Low Dose Naltrexone in Opioid Detoxification: A Double-Blind, Randomized Clinical Trial of Efficacy and Safety." *Toxicological Research* 36 (1): 21–27. https://link.springer.com/article/10.1007/s43188-019-00008-2.

– Alexander, Walter. 2012. "2012 Integrative Healthcare Symposium: Treating the Pain of Lyme Disease and Adopting Lifestyle Change as Therapy." *Pharmacy and Therapeutics* 37 (4): 247. https://pmc.ncbi.nlm.nih.gov/articles/PMC3351864/

– American Psychiatric Association. 2022. "Diagnostic and Statistical Manual of Mental Disorders." *Diagnostic and Statistical Manual of Mental Disorders*, Fifth Edition, Text Revision (DSM-5-TR) 5 (5). https://doi.org/10.1176/appi.books.9780890425787.

– Ang, Lynn, Mamta Jaiswal, Catherine Martin, and Rodica Pop-Busui. 2014. "Glucose Control and Diabetic Neuropathy: Lessons from Recent Large Clinical Trials." *Current Diabetes Reports* 14 (9). https://link.springer.com/article/10.1007/s11892-014-0528-7.

– Anne Marie McKenzie-Brown, et al., 2023. "Low-Dose Naltrexone (LDN) for Chronic Pain at a Single Institution: A Case Series." *Journal of Pain Research Volume* 16 (June): 1993–98. https://doi.org/10.2147/jpr.s389957.

– Annelyn Torres-Reverón, et al., 2016. "Endometriosis Is Associated with a Shift in MU Opioid and NMDA Receptor Expression in the Brain Periaqueductal Gray." *Reproductive Sciences* (Thousand Oaks, Calif.) 23 (9): 1158–67. https://link.springer.com/article/10.1177/1933719116630410.

– Arumugham, Vijay B., and Appaji Rayi. 2023. "Intravenous Immunoglobulin (IVIG)." PubMed. Treasure Island (FL): StatPearls Publishing. 2023. https://www.ncbi.nlm.nih.gov/books/NBK554446/.

– Banerjee, Manasi, Santanu Pal, Biswamit Bhattacharya, et al., 2013. "A Comparative Study of Efficacy and Safety of Gabapentin versus Amitriptyline as Coanalgesics in Patients Receiving Opioid Analgesics for Neuropathic Pain in Malignancy." *Indian Journal of Pharmacology* 45 (4): 334. https://doi.org/10.4103/0253-7613.115000.

– Beecher, Henry K. 1946. "Pain in Men Wounded in Battle." *Annals of Surgery* 123 (1): 96. https://pmc.ncbi.nlm.nih.gov/articles/PMC1803463/.

– Bendtsen, L., J. M. Zakrzewska, J. Abbott, et al., 2019. "European Academy of Neurology Guideline on Trigeminal Neuralgia." *European Journal of Neurology* 26 (6): 831–49. https://doi.org/10.1111/ene.13950.

– Beneciuk, Jason M., Steven Z. George, Charity G. Patterson, et al., 2022. "Treatment Effect Modifiers for Individuals with Acute Low Back Pain: Secondary Analysis of the TARGET Trial." *Pain* Publish Ahead of Print (May). https://journals.lww.com/pain/abstract/2023/01000/treatment_effect_modifiers_for_individuals_with.22.aspx.

– Berghoff, Walter. 2012. "Chronic Lyme Disease and Co-Infections: Differential Diagnosis." *The Open Neurology Journal* 6 (1): 158–78. https://pubmed.ncbi.nlm.nih.gov/23400696/

– Beutler, Sarah, et al., 2022. "Trauma-Related Dissociation and the Autonomic Nervous System: A Systematic Literature Review of Psychophysiological Correlates of Dissociative Experiencing in PTSD Patients." *European Journal of Psychotraumatology* 13 (2). https://www.tandfonline.com/doi/full/10.1080/20008066.2022.2132599.

– Birkinshaw, Hollie, Claire Friedrich, Peter Cole, et al., 2021. "Antidepressants for Pain Management in Adults with Chronic Pain: A Network Meta-Analysis." *Cochrane Database of Systematic Reviews*, April. https://www.cochranelibrary.com/cdsr/doi/10.1002/14651858.CD014682/full.

– Böttcher, Bettina, et al., 2017. "Impact of the Opioid System on the Reproductive Axis." *Fertility and Sterility* 108 (2): 207–13. https://doi.org/10.1016/j.fertnstert.2017.06.009.

– Bracken, K. L., Berman, M. E., McCloskey, M. S., & Bullock, J. S. (2008). "Deliberate Self-Harm and State Dissociation: An Experimental Investigation." *Journal of Aggression, Maltreatment & Trauma*, 17(4), 520–532. https://www.tandfonline.com/doi/abs/10.1080/10926770802463230

– Bremner, J. D., & Brett, E. (1997). "Trauma-Related Dissociative States and Long-Term Psychopathology in Posttraumatic Stress Disorder." *Journal of Traumatic Stress*, 10(1), 37–49. https://doi.org/10.1023/A:1024804312978

– Bonds, Rana S., and Terumi Midoro-Horiuti. 2013. "Estrogen Effects in Allergy and Asthma." *Current Opinion in Allergy & Clinical Immunology* 13 (1): 92–99. https://pubmed.ncbi.nlm.nih.gov/23090385/

– Bruno et al., 2018. "Targeting Toll-like Receptor-4 (TLR4)—an Emerging Therapeutic Target for Persistent Pain States." *Pain* 159 (10): 1908–15. https://journals.lww.com/pain/abstract/2018/10000/targeting_toll_like_receptor_4__tlr4__an_emerging.3.aspx.

– Burns, J. W., Bruehl, S., Chung, O. Y., et al., (2009). "Endogenous Opioids May Buffer Effects of Anger Arousal on Sensitivity To Subsequent Pain." *Pain,* 146(3), 276–282. https://journals.lww.com/pain/abstract/2009/12050/endogenous_opioids_may_buffer_effects_of_anger.12.aspx

– Butler, David S, and G Lorimer Moseley. 2018. Explain Pain. Adelaide, Australia: Noigroup Publications.

– Carvalho, Jozélio Freire de, and Thelma Skare. "Low-Dose Naltrexone in Rheumatological Diseases." *Mediterranean Journal of Rheumatology* 34, no. 1 (March 31, 2023): 1–6. https://www.mjrheum.org/assets/files/792/file429_1703.pdf.

– Castellano, C., & Puglisi-Allegra, S. (1982). "Effects of Naloxone and Naltrexone on Locomotor Activity in C57BL/6 and DBA/2 Mice." *Pharmacology, Biochemistry and Behavior,* 16(4),

561–563. https://www.sciencedirect.com/science/article/abs/pii/0091305782904154?via%3Dihub

– Chan, Michael D., Edward G. Shaw, and Stephen B. Tatter. 2013. "Radiosurgical Management of Trigeminal Neuralgia." *Neurosurgery Clinics of North America* 24 (4): 613–21. https://doi.org/10.1016/j.nec.2013.05.001.

– Chopra, Pradeep et al., 2017. "Pain Management in the Ehlers-Danlos Syndromes." *American Journal of Medical Genetics Part C: Seminars in Medical Genetics* 175 (1): 212–19. https://onlinelibrary.wiley.com/doi/10.1002/ajmg.c.31554.

– Chopra, Pradeep, and Mark S. Cooper. 2013. "Treatment of Complex Regional Pain Syndrome (CRPS) Using Low Dose Naltrexone (LDN)." *Journal of Neuroimmune Pharmacology* 8 (3): 470–76. https://link.springer.com/article/10.1007/s11481-013-9451-y

– Christopher Theriault, Omonike Oyelola, and William T Zempsky, "The Efficacy of Low-Dose Naltrexone in Pediatric Chronic Pain: A Retrospective Analysis," *The Journal of Pain* 24, no. 4 (April 1, 2023): 84–85, https://doi.org/10.1016/j.jpain.2023.02.243

– Clauw, Daniel J. 2014. "Fibromyalgia: A Clinical Review." *JAMA* 311 (15): 1547. https://jamanetwork.com/journals/jama/article-abstract/1860480.

– Coventry, P. A., Meader, N., Melton, H., et al., (2020). "Psychological and Pharmacological Interventions for Posttraumatic Stress Disorder and Comorbid Mental Health Problems Following Complex Traumatic Events: Systematic Review and Component Network Meta-Analysis." *PLoS Medicine*, 17(8), e1003262. https://journals.plos.org/plosmedicine/article?id=10.1371/journal.pmed.1003262

– Dara, Praneet. "Opiate Antagonists for Chronic Pain: A Review on the Benefits of Low-Dose Naltrexone in Arthritis versus Non-Arthritic Diseases." *Biomedicines* 11, no. 6 (June 1, 2023): 1620. https://doi.org/10.3390/biomedicines11061620.

– Dijana Hadžiomerović-Pekić, et al., 2010. "Metformin, Naltrexone, or the Combination of Prednisolone and Antiandrogenic Oral Contraceptives as First-Line Therapy in Hyperinsulinemic Women with Polycystic Ovary Syndrome." *Fertility and Sterility* 94 (6): 2385–88. https://doi.org/10.1016/j.fertnstert.2010.02.041.

– Driver, C. Noelle, and Ryan S. D'Souza. 2023. "Efficacy of Low-Dose Naltrexone and Predictors of Treatment Success or Discontinuation in Fibromyalgia and Other Chronic Pain Conditions: A Fourteen-Year, Enterprise-Wide Retrospective Analysis." *Biomedicines* 11 (4): 1087. https://www.mdpi.com/2227-9059/11/4/1087.

– Dupont, John S. 2003. "The Prevalence of Trigeminal Neuritis with TMD." *CRANIO®* 21 (3): 180–84. https://www.tandfonline.com/doi/abs/10.1080/08869634.2003.11746248.

– Eisenlohr-Moul, et al., 2017. "Toward the Reliable Diagnosis of DSM-5 Premenstrual Dysphoric Disorder: The Carolina Premenstrual Assessment Scoring System (C-PASS)." *American Journal of Psychiatry* 174 (1): 51–59. https://psychiatryonline.org/doi/10.1176/appi.ajp.2016.15121510

– EMDR International Association. 2024. "Neurobiology and Treatment of Traumatic Dissociation: Towards an Embodied Self (Springer, 2014)." *EMDR International Association.* August 26, 2024. https://www.emdria.org/resource/neurobiology-and-treatment-of-traumatic-dissociation-towards-and-embodied-self-springer-2014/.

– Escamilla, Irene et al., "Treatment of Dissociative Symptoms with Opioid Antagonists: A Systematic Review." *European Journal of Psychotraumatology* 14, no. 2 (2023): 2265184. https://www.tandfonline.com/doi/full/10.1080/20008066.2023.2265184.

– EULAR Textbook on the Rheumatic Diseases; Editor Johannes WJ Bijlsma; 2012; BMJ Group

– Fabbri, A., E.A. Jannini, L. Gnessi, et al., 1989. "Endorphins in Male Impotence: Evidence for Naltrexone Stimulation of Erectile Activity in Patient Therapy." *Psychoneuroendocrinology* 14 (1-2): 103–11. https://doi.org/10.1016/0306-4530(89)90059-0.

– Fechir, M., Breimhorst, M., Kritzmann, S., et al., (2012). "Naloxone Inhibits Not Only Stress-Induced Analgesia but also Sympathetic Activation and Baroreceptor-Reflex Sensitivity." *European Journal of*

Pain (London, England), 16(1), 82–92. https://onlinelibrary.wiley.com/doi/10.1016/j.ejpain.2011.06.009

– Fink, M., et al., 2009. "Catatonia Is Not Schizophrenia: Kraepelin's Error and the Need to Recognize Catatonia as an Independent Syndrome in Medical Nomenclature." *Schizophrenia Bulletin* 36 (2): 314–20. https://academic.oup.com/schizophreniabulletin/article-abstract/36/2/314/1899222?redirectedFrom=fulltext.

– Gara, Soumaya et al., 2023. "Juvenile Dermatomyositis." StatPearls, Winter. https://pubmed.ncbi.nlm.nih.gov/30480969/.

– Girach, Ayesha, Thomas Henry Julian, Giustino Varrassi, et al., 2019. "Quality of Life in Painful Peripheral Neuropathies: A Systematic Review." *Pain Research and Management* 2019 (May): 1–9. https://doi.org/10.1155/2019/2091960.

– Grichnik, K.P. And Ferrante, F.M., 1991 "The Difference between Acute and Chronic Pain." *The Mount Sinai Journal of Medicine*, 58, 217-220. - References - Scientific Research Publishing." 2018. Scirp.org. 2018. https://www.scirp.org/reference/referencespapers?referenceid=2214256.

– Groman, Stephanie M., Bart Massi, Samuel R. Mathias, Daeyeol Lee, and Jane R. Taylor. 2019. "Model-Free and Model-Based Influences in Addiction-Related Behaviors." *Biological Psychiatry* 85 (11): 936–45. https://doi.org/10.1016/j.biopsych.2018.12.017.

– Hamed, Khalid M et al., 2022. "Overview of Methotrexate Toxicity: A Comprehensive Literature Review." *Cureus* 14 (9). https://www.cureus.com/articles/114596-overview-of-methotrexate-toxicity-a-comprehensive-literature-review#!/.

– Haney, Margaret, Adam Bisaga, and Richard W. Foltin. 2003. "Interaction between Naltrexone and Oral THC in Heavy Marijuana Smokers." *Psychopharmacology* 166 (1): 77–85. https://link.springer.com/article/10.1007/s00213-002-1279-8.

– Harden, R. Norman, et al., 2007. "Proposed New Diagnostic Criteria for Complex Regional Pain Syndrome." *Pain Medicine* 8 (4): 326–31. https://

academic.oup.com/painmedicine/article-abstract/8/4/326/1818293?redire
ctedFrom=fulltext.

– Häuser, Winfried, Brian Walitt, Mary-Ann Fitzcharles, and Claudia
Sommer. 2014. "Review of Pharmacological Therapies in Fibromyalgia
Syndrome." *Arthritis Research & Therapy* 16 (1): 201. https://doi.
org/10.1186/ar4441.

– Holbech, Jakob Vormstrup, Anne Jung, Torsten Jonsson, Mette Wanning,
Claus Bredahl, and Flemming Bach. 2017. "Combination Treatment of
Neuropathic Pain: Danish Expert Recommendations Based on a Delphi
Process." *Journal of Pain Research* Volume 10 (June): 1467–75. https://
doi.org/10.2147/jpr.s138099.

– Horowitz, Richard I. and Phyllis R. Freeman. 2018. "Precision Medicine:
The Role of the MSIDS Model in Defining, Diagnosing, and Treating
Chronic Lyme Disease/Post Treatment Lyme Disease Syndrome and
Other Chronic Illness: Part 2." *Healthcare* 6 (4): 129. https://www.mdpi.
com/2227-9032/6/4/129

– Huang, Lang, et al., 2017. "Opioid-Induced Constipation Relief from
Fixed-Ratio Combination Prolonged-Release Oxycodone/Naloxone
Compared with Oxycodone and Morphine for Chronic Nonmalignant
Pain: A Systematic Review and Meta-Analysis of Randomized Controlled
Trials." *Journal of Pain and Symptom Management* 54 (5): 737-748.e3.
https://doi.org/10.1016/j.jpainsymman.2017.07.025.

– Jarred Younger et al., "Low-Dose Naltrexone for the Treatment of
Fibromyalgia: Findings of a Small, Randomized, Double-Blind, Placebo-
Controlled, Counterbalanced, Crossover Trial Assessing Daily Pain
Levels," *Arthritis and Rheumatism* 65, no. 2 (2013): 529–38, https://doi.
org/10.1002/art.37734.

– Jarred Younger, Luke Parkitny, and David McLain, "The Use of Low-
Dose Naltrexone (LDN) as a Novel Anti-Inflammatory Treatment for
Chronic Pain," *Clinical Rheumatology* 33, no. 4 (February 15, 2014):
451–59, https://link.springer.com/article/10.1007/s10067-014-2517-2.

– Joanna Jaros and Peter Lio, "Low Dose Naltrexone in Dermatology," *Journal of Drugs in Dermatology*: JDD 18, no. 3 (March 1, 2019): 235–38, https://pubmed.ncbi.nlm.nih.gov/30909326/

– Johnson, B. N., McKernan, L. C., & Bruehl, S. (2022). "A Theoretical Endogenous Opioid Neurobiological Framework for Co-occurring Pain, Trauma, and Non-suicidal Self-Injury." *Current Pain and Headache Reports*, 26(6), 405–414. https://link.springer.com/article/10.1007/s11916-022-01043-9

– Karlo Toljan and Bruce Vrooman, "Low-Dose Naltrexone (LDN)—Review of Therapeutic Utilization," *Medical Sciences* 6, no. 4 (September 21, 2018): 82, https://www.mdpi.com/2076-3271/6/4/82.

– Kim, P. S., & Fishman, M. A. (2020). "Low-Dose Naltrexone for Chronic Pain: Update and Systemic Review." *Current Pain and Headache Reports,* 24(10), 64. https://link.springer.com/article/10.1007/s11916-020-00898-0

– Kozlowska, K., Walker, P., McLean, L., & Carrive, P. (2015). "Fear and the Defense Cascade: Clinical Implications and Management." *Harvard Review of Psychiatry*, 23(4), 263–287. https://journals.lww.com/hrpjournal/fulltext/2015/07000/fear_and_the_defense_cascade__clinical.3.aspx

– Kučić N, Rački V, Šverko R, Vidović T, Grahovac I, Mršić-Pelčić J. "Immunometabolic Modulatory Role of Naltrexone in BV-2 Microglia Cells." *International Journal of Molecular Sciences*. 2021 Aug 5;22(16):8429. https://pubmed.ncbi.nlm.nih.gov/34445130/

– Lanius, Ruth A., et al., 2018. "A Review of the Neurobiological Basis of Trauma-Related Dissociation and Its Relation to Cannabinoid- and Opioid-Mediated Stress Response: A Transdiagnostic, Translational Approach." *Current Psychiatry Reports* 20 (12). https://link.springer.com/article/10.1007/s11920-018-0983-y.

– Lanius, Ulrich and Forster, Galyn, "The LDN Book, Volume Two," Chelsea Green Publishing, July 11, 2020, Chapter 10, https://www.chelseagreen.com/product/the-ldn-book-volume-two/?srsltid=AfmBOoqu7QY4aSfxyf4tkJdEY7YxLDMg8tnyLr3EuYUtOwziwXU2kZ2f.

– Lanius, Ulrich F et al., "Neurobiology and Treatment of Traumatic Dissociation: Toward an Embodied Self," New York: Springer Publishing Company, 2014.

– Latremoliere, Alban, and Clifford J. Woolf. 2009. "Central Sensitization: A Generator of Pain Hypersensitivity by Central Neural Plasticity." *The Journal of Pain* 10 (9): 895–926. https://doi.org/10.1016/j. jpain.2009.06.012.

– Lefaucheur, Jean-Pascal, et al., 2020. "Evidence-Based Guidelines on the Therapeutic Use of Repetitive Transcranial Magnetic Stimulation (RTMS): An Update (2014–2018)." *Clinical Neurophysiology* 131 (2): 474–528. https://doi.org/10.1016/j.clinph.2019.11.002

– Li, Z., You, Y., Griffin, N., Feng, J. and Shan, F. (2018). "Low-dose Naltrexone (LDN): A Promising Treatment in Immune-Related Diseases and Cancer Therapy." *International Immunopharmacology*, 61, pp.178–184. https://doi.org/10.1016/j.intimp.2018.05.020.

– Longden, Eleanor, et al., 2020. "The Relationship between Dissociation and Symptoms of Psychosis: A Meta-Analysis." *Schizophrenia Bulletin* 46 (5): 1104–13. https://academic.oup.com/schizophreniabulletin/article-abst ract/46/5/1104/5816610?redirectedFrom=fulltext.

– Mahgoub, Yassir, et al., 2024. "Catatonia and Melancholia Interface: Exploring a New Paradigm for Evaluation and Treatment. A Case Series and Literature Review." *Frontiers in Psychiatry* 15 (March). https://www. frontiersin.org/journals/psychiatry/articles/10.3389/fpsyt.2024.1372136/ full.

– Majuri, Joonas et al., "Dopamine and Opioid Neurotransmission in Behavioral Addictions: A Comparative PET Study in Pathological Gambling and Binge Eating." *Neuropsychopharmacology* 42, no. 5 (November 24, 2016): 1169–77. https://doi.org/10.1038/npp.2016.265.

– Malfait, Fransiska, et al. 2020. "The Ehlers–Danlos Syndromes." *Nature Reviews Disease Primers* 6 (1). https://doi.org/10.1038/s41572-020-0194-9.

– Marcus, Norman J., et al., 2024. "Effective Doses of Low-Dose Naltrexone for Chronic Pain - an Observational Study." *Journal of Pain Research* 17: 1273–84. https://doi.org/10.2147/JPR.S451183.

– Maercker, A., Cloitre, M., Bachem, R. et al., (2022). "Complex Post-Traumatic Stress Disorder." *Lancet* (London, England), 400(10345), 60–72.   https://www.thelancet.com/journals/lancet/article/PIIS0140-6736(22)00821-2/abstract

– McKenzie-Brown, et al., 2021. "Low-Dose Naltrexone in Endometrial Intraepithelial Neoplasia." *Pain Medicine* 23 (4): 866–68. https://doi.org/10.1093/pm/pnab212.

– McLaughlin, Patricia J, Ian S Zagon, et al., 2009. "Growth Inhibition of Thyroid Follicular Cell-Derived Cancers by the Opioid Growth Factor (OGF) - Opioid Growth Factor Receptor (OGFr) Axis." *BMC Cancer* 9 (1). https://bmccancer.biomedcentral.com/articles/10.1186/1471-2407-9-369.

– Meglathery MD: RCCX Theory Explains Overlapping Medical and Psychiatric Syndromes Associated with Chronic Illness, PART I." 2015. Meglathery MD: Coinherited CYP21A2, TNXB, C4 Genes in Chronic Illness (CFS, FM, Lyme, MCAS, POTS, Pain, Psychiatric Spectrum, Immunological, Endocrine) +- Hypermobility +- Autoimmune Diseases. 2015.   https://www.rccxandillness.com/rccx-theory-part-i-genes-and-properties-of-the-rccx-module-explain-clusters-of-illness-in-families-and-all-the-symptomssyndromes-found-in-chronic-illness.html.

– Marcus, Norman J., Lexi Robbins, et al., 2024. "Effective Doses of Low-Dose Naltrexone for Chronic Pain - an Observational Study." *Journal of Pain Research* 17: 1273–84. https://pubmed.ncbi.nlm.nih.gov/38532991/

– Mikus, Nace et al., "Effects of Dopamine D2/3 and Opioid Receptor Antagonism on the Trade-off between Model-Based and Model-Free Behaviour in Healthy Volunteers." *ELife* 11 (December 5, 2022): e79661. https://doi.org/10.7554/eLife.79661.

– Miller, M. W., Lin, A. P., Wolf, E. J., & Miller, D. R. (2018). "Oxidative Stress, Inflammation, and Neuroprogression in Chronic PTSD." *Harvard Review of Psychiatry*, 26(2), 57–69. https://journals.lww.com/hrpjournal/abstract/2018/03000/oxidative_stress,_inflammation,_and.2.aspx

– Mischoulon, David. "Randomized, Proof-of-Concept Trial of Low Dose Naltrexone for Patients with Breakthrough Symptoms of Major Depressive Disorder on Antidepressants." *Journal of Affective Disorders* 208 (January 2017): 6–14. https://doi.org/10.1016/j.jad.2016.08.029.

– Mosch, Benjamin et al., 2023. "Brain Morphometric Changes in Fibromyalgia and the Impact of Psychometric and Clinical Factors: A Volumetric and Diffusion-Tensor Imaging Study", 25 (1), *Arthritis Research & Therapy*. https://arthritis-research.biomedcentral.com/articles/10.1186/s13075-023-03064-0.

– Norman Brown, Jaak Panksepp, "Low-dose Naltrexone for Disease Prevention and Quality of Life," *Medical Hypotheses* 72(3), (March 2009): 333-7, https://pubmed.ncbi.nlm.nih.gov/19041189/

– Ostacher, M. J., & Cifu, A. S. (2019). "Management of Posttraumatic Stress Disorder." *JAMA*, 321(2), 200–201. https://jamanetwork.com/journals/jama/article-abstract/2719367

– Panksepp, J., & Biven, L. (2012). The archaeology of mind: Neuroevolutionary origins of human emotion. W. W. Norton & Company.

– Paolo Mannelli, Ashwin A Patkar, Kathleen Peindl, et al., 2009. "Early Outcomes Following Low Dose Naltrexone Enhancement of Opioid Detoxification." *American Journal on Addictions* 18 (2): 109–16. https://doi.org/10.1080/10550490902772785.

– Pape, W. and Wöller, W., "Niedrig Dosiertes Naltrexon in Der Behandlung Dissoziativer Symptome." *Der Nervenarzt* 86, no. 3 (2015): 346–51. https://link.springer.com/article/10.1007/s00115-014-4015-9.

– Paquette, Jay, and Mary Olmstead. 2005. "Ultra-Low Dose Naltrexone Enhances Cannabinoid-Induced Antinociception." *Behavioural Pharmacology* 16 (8): 597–603. https://journals.lww.com/behaviouralpharm/abstract/2005/12000/ultra_low_dose_naltrexone_enhances.1.aspx.

– Patten, Denise K., et al., 2018. "The Safety and Efficacy of Low-Dose Naltrexone in the Management of Chronic Pain and Inflammation in Multiple Sclerosis, Fibromyalgia, Crohn's Disease, and Other Chronic Pain Disorders." *Pharmacotherapy: The Journal of Human Pharmacology*

and Drug Therapy 38 (3): 382–89. https://accpjournals.onlinelibrary.
wiley.com/doi/10.1002/phar.2086.

– Phillip S. Kim and Michael A. Fishman, "Low-Dose Naltrexone for
Chronic Pain: Update and Systemic Review," *Current Pain and Headache
Reports* 24, no. 10 (August 26, 2020), https://doi.org/10.1007/s11916-
020-00898-0.

– Raknes, Guttorm, and Lars Småbrekke. "Low Dose Naltrexone: Effects
on Medication in Rheumatoid and Seropositive Arthritis. A Nationwide
Register-Based Controlled Quasi-Experimental Before-after Study."
PLOS ONE 14, no. 2 (February 14, 2019): e0212460. https://journals.plos.
org/plosone/article?id=10.1371/journal.pone.0212460.

– Rodriguez-Iturbe, Bernardo, Hector Pons, and Richard J. Johnson. 2017.
"Role of the Immune System in Hypertension." *Physiological Reviews* 97
(3): 1127–64. https://doi.org/10.1152/physrev.00031.2016.

– Roelofs, Karin. 2017. "Freeze for Action: Neurobiological Mechanisms
in Animal and Human Freezing." *Philosophical Transactions of
the Royal Society B: Biological Sciences* 372 (1718). https://
royalsocietypublishing.org/doi/10.1098/rstb.2016.0206

– Roelofs, K., & Dayan, P. (2022). "Freezing Revisited: Coordinated
Autonomic and Central Optimization of Threat Coping." *Nature Reviews.
Neuroscience*, 23(9), 568–580. https://www.nature.com/articles/s41583-
022-00608-2

– Rosebush, P. I., and M. F. Mazurek. 2009. "Catatonia and Its Treatment."
Schizophrenia Bulletin 36 (2): 239–42. https://doi.org/10.1093/schbul/
sbp141.

– Rosenblum, Michael D. et al., 2015. "Mechanisms of Human
Autoimmunity." *Journal of Clinical Investigation* 125 (6): 2228–33.
https://www.jci.org/articles/view/78088.

– Rupp, Adam et al., 2023. "Low Dose Naltrexone's Utility for Non-Cancer
Centralized Pain Conditions - a Scoping Review." *Pain Medicine*, June.
https://academic.oup.com/painmedicine/article/24/11/1270/7193901.

– Sadee, Wolfgang, and John C McKew. 2022. "Ligand-Free Signaling
of G-Protein-Coupled Receptors: Relevance to μ Opioid Receptors in

Analgesia and Addiction." *Molecules* (Basel, Switzerland) 27 (18). https://www.mdpi.com/1420-3049/27/18/5826.

– Sadee, Wolfgang, et al., 2020. "Biased Opioid Antagonists as Modulators of Opioid Dependence: Opportunities to Improve Pain Therapy and Opioid Use Management." *Molecules* 25 (18). https://www.mdpi.com/1420-3049/25/18/4163.

– Sarkar, P., et al., 2004. "Dissociative Disorder Presenting as Catatonia." *Indian Journal of Psychiatry* 46 (2): 176–79. https://pubmed.ncbi.nlm.nih.gov/21408047/.

– Scaer, R. C. (2001). "The Body Bears the Burden: Trauma, Dissociation, and Disease." Haworth Press.

– Schore, Allan, "The Effects of Early Relational Trauma on Right Brain Development, Affect Regulation, and Infant Mental Health," *Infant Mental Health Journal* 22, no. 1-2 (2001): 201–69, https://www.allanschore.com/pdf/SchoreIMHJTrauma01.pdf.

– Sène, Damien. 2018. "Small Fiber Neuropathy: Diagnosis, Causes, and Treatment." *Joint Bone Spine* 85 (5): 553–59. https://doi.org/10.1016/j.jbspin.2017.11.002.

– Sharp, Madeleine E. et al., "Dopamine Selectively Remediates 'Model-Based' Reward Learning: A Computational Approach." *Brain* 139, no. 2 (December 17, 2015): 355–64. https://academic.oup.com/brain/article/139/2/355/1753805.

– Spencer CN, Elton A, Dove S, et al., "Naltrexone Engages a Brain Reward Network in the Presence of Reward-Predictive Distractor Stimuli in Males." *Addiction Neuroscience.* 2023 Sep;7:100085 . https://pmc.ncbi.nlm.nih.gov/articles/PMC10328541/

– Teicher, M. H., Samson, J. A., Anderson, et al., (2016). "The Effects of Childhood Maltreatment on Brain Structure, Function and Connectivity." *Nature reviews. Neuroscience*, 17(10), 652–666. https://www.nature.com/articles/nrn.2016.111

– Tesarz, Jonas, et al., 2019. "EMDR Therapy's Efficacy in the Treatment of Pain." *Journal of EMDR Practice and Research* 13 (4): 337–44. https://connect.springerpub.com/content/sgremdr/13/4/337.

– "The Escalation of the Opioid Epidemic due to COVID-19 and Resulting Lessons about Treatment Alternatives." 2020. *The American Journal of Managed Care* 26 (7): e202–4. https://doi.org/10.37765/ajmc.2020.43386.

– Theriault, Christopher, Omonike Oyelola, and William T Zempsky. 2023. "The Efficacy of Low-Dose Naltrexone in Pediatric Chronic Pain: A Retrospective Analysis." The Journal of Pain 24 (4): 84–85. https://www.jpain.org/article/S1526-5900(23)00282-1/fulltext

– Tidd, Samantha J. Stallkamp, Christopher Cantrell, Brady D. Greene, et al., 2023. "Low-Dose Naltrexone Use in Postural Orthostatic Tachycardia Syndrome: A Case Series." *Cureus* 15 (8). https://www.cureus.com/articles/176869-low-dose-naltrexone-use-in-postural-orthostatic-tachycardia-syndrome-a-case-series#!/.

– Timäus, Charles et al., "Efficacy of Naltrexone in Borderline Personality Disorder, a Retrospective Analysis in Inpatients." *Human Psychopharmacology: Clinical and Experimental*, May 24, 2021. https://onlinelibrary.wiley.com/doi/10.1002/hup.2800.

– Voon, Valerie et al., "The Neurochemical Substrates of Habitual and Goal-Directed Control" 10, no. 1 (March 3, 2020). https://doi.org/10.1038/s41398-020-0762-5.

– Wardle, M. C., Bershad, A. K., & de Wit, H. (2016). "Naltrexone Alters the Processing of Social and Emotional Stimuli in Healthy Adults." *Social Neuroscience*, 11(6), 579–591. https://www.tandfonline.com/doi/full/10.1080/17470919.2015.1136355

– Watkins, Linda R., et al., 2001. "Glial Activation: A Driving Force for Pathological Pain." *Trends in Neurosciences* 24 (8): 450–55. https://www.cell.com/trends/neurosciences/abstract/S0166-2236(00)01854-3?_returnURL=https%3A%2F%2Flinkinghub.elsevier.com%2Fretrieve%2Fpii%2FS0166223600018543%3Fshowall%3Dtrue.

– Weinstock LB, et al., "Low-Dose Naltrexone Therapy for Psoriasis," *International Journal of Pharmaceutical Compounding* 24(2) (March 1, 2020): 94-96, https://europepmc.org/article/med/32196470

– Weinstock, Leonard B., Renee M. Nelson, and Svetlana Blitshteyn. 2023. "Neuropsychiatric Manifestations of Mast Cell Activation Syndrome and

Response to Mast-Cell-Directed Treatment: A Case Series." *Journal of Personalized Medicine* 13 (11): 1562. https://pubmed.ncbi.nlm.nih.gov/38003876/

– Weinstock, Leonard B., Jill B. Brook, et al., 2021. "Mast Cell Activation Symptoms Are Prevalent in Long-COVID." *International Journal of Infectious Diseases* 112 (September). https://pubmed.ncbi.nlm.nih.gov/34563706/

– Weinstock, Leonard B., Jill Brook, et al., 2019. "Small Intestinal Bacterial Overgrowth Is Common in Mast Cell Activation Syndrome." *American Journal of Gastroenterology* 114 (1): S671–71. https://scivisionpub.com/pdfs/small-intestinal-bacterial-overgrowth-is-common-in-mast-cell-activation-syndrome-1371.pdf

– Weinstock, Leonard B., Jill B. Brook, Trisha L. Myers, and Brent Goodman. 2018. "Successful Treatment of Postural Orthostatic Tachycardia and Mast Cell Activation Syndromes Using Naltrexone, Immunoglobulin and Antibiotic Treatment." *BMJ Case Reports* 2018 (January): bcr2017221405, bcr–2017-221405. https://pubmed.ncbi.nlm.nih.gov/29326369/

– Winters, Bryony L., Gabrielle C. Gregoriou, Sarah A. Kissiwaa, et al., 2017. "Endogenous Opioids Regulate Moment-To-Moment Neuronal Communication and Excitability." *Nature Communications* 8 (1): 14611. https://www.nature.com/articles/ncomms14611.

– Zagon, Ian S, and Patricia J McLaughlin. 2018. "Intermittent Blockade of OGFr and Treatment of Autoimmune Disorders." *Experimental Biology and Medicine* 243 (17-18): 1323–30. https://journals.sagepub.com/doi/10.1177/1535370218817746.

Index

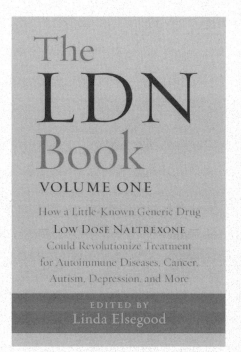

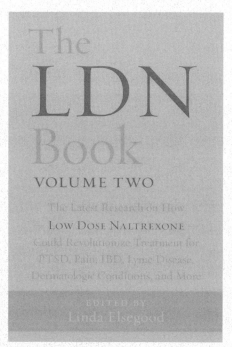

The LDN Book's Volume 1 & Volume 2 Published by Chelsea Green Publishing

The Books in the LDN Series

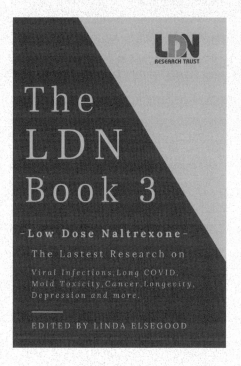

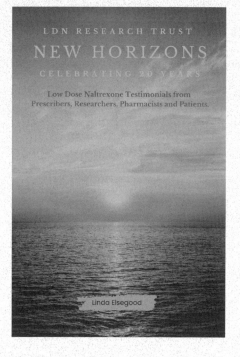

The LDN Book 3 & New Horizons Published by The LDN Research Trust

About The Editor

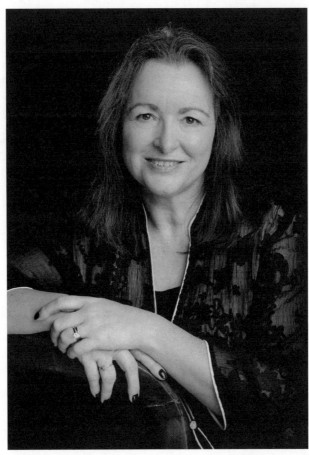

Photo by Julia Holland

Linda Elsegood is the founder of LDN Research Trust, a UK charity created in 2004. Living with Multiple Sclerosis (MS) herself, she experienced significant benefits from low-dose naltrexone (LDN) and felt compelled to assist others not only with MS but also with various autoimmune diseases, cancers, and mental health challenges. Over the past 21 years, her charity has positively impacted the lives of more than two million individuals globally.